Praise for *A Nurse's Step-* *Dissertation*

"*Karen Roush's book is an essential resource for all nursing scholars, most notably new graduates of doctoral programs. The book breaks down the complexities of scholarly writing and provides key insight and vital guidance for publishing dissertations or DNP projects. Roush is an accomplished professor, writer, and editor who shares her expertise in writing for publication in this new book.* A Nurse's Step-by-Step Guide to Publishing a Dissertation or DNP Project *will have a permanent place on my bookshelf and will be shared with new graduates and colleagues alike.*"

–Nancy White Street, ScD, PPCNP-BC
Julia and Harold Plotnick Professor of Global Nursing
University of Massachusetts Dartmouth College of Nursing

"*It is an honor to have the opportunity to read and review Karen Roush's well-written, user-friendly guide and pearls for nursing doctoral students (PhD and DNP) to use in navigating the often-daunting world of publication. This text is an excellent supplement to faculty writing mentorship for students as they tackle preparation of their dissertation or scholarly project for dissemination. I found the differentiation between the purpose of a student paper and manuscript, the description of the iterative writing process, and specific examples of grammatical fatal flaws—as well as the 'write this, not this' tips and the submission process—to be spot on!*"

–Susan Sullivan-Bolyai, DNSc, CNS, RN, FAAN
Professor of Nursing & Pediatrics
Associate Dean for Research and Innovation
UMass Medical School-Graduate School of Nursing

"*Karen Roush's earlier book on writing a dissertation or scholarly project has become the 'go-to' resource for scores of doctoral students. In her new book,* A Nurse's Step-by-Step Guide to Publishing a Dissertation or DNP Project, *Roush has again demonstrated her unique knack for simplifying a process—the often-arduous steps necessary for turning a dissertation or capstone project into a manuscript worthy of publication. A must-read primer for anyone wanting to publish.*"

–Wendy Budin, PhD, RN-BC, FAAN
Professor & Associate Dean
Entry to Baccalaureate Practice Division
Editor-in-Chief, *Journal of Perinatal Education*
Rutgers, The State University of New Jersey
School of Nursing

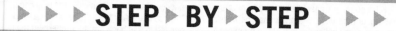

A NURSE'S

▶ ▶ ▶ **STEP** ▶ **BY** ▶ **STEP** ▶ ▶ ▶

GUIDE TO

PUBLISHING A DISSERTATION OR DNP PROJECT

TAKING YOUR PAPER FROM GRADUATION TO PUBLICATION

KAREN ROUSH, PhD, RN, FNP-BC

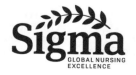

Sigma

GLOBAL NURSING
EXCELLENCE

Sigma Theta Tau International Honor Society of Nursing (Sigma) is a nonprofit organization whose mission is advancing world health and celebrating nursing excellence in scholarship, leadership, and service. Founded in 1922, Sigma has more than 135,000 active members in over 90 countries and territories. Members include practicing nurses, instructors, researchers, policymakers, entrepreneurs, and others. Sigma's more than 530 chapters are located at more than 700 institutions of higher education throughout Armenia, Australia, Botswana, Brazil, Canada, Colombia, England, Ghana, Hong Kong, Ireland, Jamaica, Japan, Jordan, Kenya, Lebanon, Malawi, Mexico, the Netherlands, Nigeria, Pakistan, Philippines, Portugal, Puerto Rico, Singapore, South Africa, South Korea, Swaziland, Sweden, Taiwan, Tanzania, Thailand, the United States, and Wales. Learn more at www.sigmanursing.org.

Sigma Theta Tau International
550 West North Street
Indianapolis, IN, USA 46202

To order additional books, buy in bulk, or order for corporate use, contact Sigma Marketplace at 888.654.4968 (US and Canada) or +1.317.634.8171 (outside US and Canada).

To request a review copy for course adoption, email solutions@sigmamarketplace.org or call 888.654.4968 (US and Canada) or +1.317.634.8171 (outside US and Canada).

To request author information, or for speaker or other media requests, contact Sigma Marketing at 888.634.7575 (US and Canada) or +1.317.634.8171 (outside US and Canada).

ISBN: 9781948057370
EPUB ISBN: 9781948057387
PDF ISBN: 9781948057394
MOBI ISBN: 9781948057400

Library of Congress Cataloging-in-Publication data

LCCN Permalink: https://lccn.loc.gov/2019021732

First Printing, 2019

Publisher: Dustin Sullivan
Acquisitions Editor: Emily Hatch
Development Editor: Carla Hall
Cover Designer: Rebecca Batchelor
Interior Design/Page Layout: Rebecca Batchelor

Managing Editor: Carla Hall
Project Editor: Todd Lothery
Copy Editor: Gill Editorial Services
Proofreaders: Jane Palmer and Todd Lothery
Indexer: Larry D. Sweazy

Dedication

This book is dedicated to the *AJN* crew for sharing their friendship and writing talents with me. You've enriched my writing and my life.

About the Author

Karen Roush, PhD, RN, FNP-BC, received her PhD in nursing research and theory development from the New York University Rory Meyers College of Nursing. She started her nursing education with an associate degree in nursing from Adirondack Community College in 1982, went on for her BSN at Russell Sage College, and then earned a master's degree at Columbia University, where she specialized as a family nurse practitioner.

Roush served for many years as Editorial Director and Clinical Managing Editor for the *American Journal of Nursing (AJN)* and continues her affiliation with the journal as News Director. In addition, she is the founder of The Scholar's Voice, which works to strengthen the voice of nursing through writing mentorship for nurses. In this capacity, Roush works with nurses in varied roles, including doctoral students, faculty members, nursing leaders, and bedside nurses. She is particularly proud of her success working with bedside nurses and other novice writers and shares their joy when they become published authors for the first time. She is an award-winning writer who has authored multiple consumer health-care books, numerous nursing articles in peer-reviewed journals, essays, and poetry. Roush has traveled to Rwanda, Uganda, and India as a nursing volunteer and taught nursing students in Ghana. She was a visiting scholar in the Department of Human Resources for Health at the World Health Organization in Geneva, Switzerland. Currently she works as adjunct faculty at Pace University and The Graduate Center for the City University of New York.

Table of Contents

Introduction: Becoming an Author

It's time to share your work with the world.

In the Introduction of your dissertation or project paper, you told your committee why your research or project was important. You persuaded them that this was a topic or problem that we needed to pay attention to. But if only your committee members have paid attention, the impact ends there. Don't let what you've accomplished sit in the bottom of a drawer or in a fancy binder on a shelf. Make sure it gets to the people who can use it—other nurses who are struggling to solve the same problems you've addressed; clinicians who need evidence to provide the highest quality, most effective care; researchers building a body of knowledge; and nursing leaders trying to influence policy at local and national levels.

Perhaps you've presented your project and its outcomes to your colleagues and leadership in your organization. Maybe they've even taken it beyond your unit and created a facility-wide protocol based on what you did. Or you've presented your research at a conference where you shared it with a few hundred attendees. People came up to talk to you after a podium presentation or stopped by your poster.

Those presentations are important and are effective in disseminating your results to others interested in your topic. They may even result in replication of your project or collaborations with other researchers. But they don't have the reach of publication. When you publish your work in a respected journal, it has the potential to reach thousands. Your research will become part of the body of knowledge—a building block of nursing science. The project you undertook to improve the care of patients on one unit or in one facility now has the potential to improve care for an untold number of patients everywhere.

Publishing the results of your dissertation or scholarly project is the final step in your doctoral education process. No, your dissertation or project was not your life's work, but neither was it just another student exercise. It was a meaningful endeavor that asked others—participants, key stakeholders, mentors—to contribute their time and effort and expertise. You owe it to them, to future patients, and to nursing science to share what you learned through your work.

Negative findings. You should still publish your dissertation or project if your hypotheses were not proven or your project didn't result in the outcomes you hoped for. Knowing what doesn't work—and why—is important so others don't waste time and resources researching questions you've already answered or hitting the same barriers you've encountered. Unlike in the past, many journals now recognize the importance of publishing reports of negative findings.

Publication is powerful. Research enables you to influence nursing practice and patient outcomes far beyond your corner of the world. The lives of people you will never meet may be better because of your work. Publication connects you to people with similar interests, experiences, and goals. Or it ignites a curiosity in people who weren't interested before. And they go on to build on what you've contributed. It ensures that what you believe needs to be paid attention to *is* paid attention to.

Publication is also important because it strengthens the voice of nursing in the healthcare arena. It is our responsibility to make sure that nursing work—the entire breadth and depth of it—is made visible. There is still a lack of awareness of the contributions that nurses make to science, healthcare policy, clinical practice decisions, and healthcare systems design and management.

Writing a high-quality manuscript is difficult. It takes a lot of focused time and effort to take a paper from a first draft to a publishable manuscript. And turning a long, complex dissertation or project paper into a concise, focused manuscript presents its own set of challenges. You will get frustrated along the way. When you produce just one page of decent writing after spending hours at your computer, you'll question yourself. You'll think maybe you're just not good at this writing stuff. Not true. Good writing takes critical thinking, reflection, and circling back again and again to make sure everything is connected, logical, accurate, and clearly written. All that takes time.

And you've had a lot of practice writing throughout your doctoral program. You've read tons of scholarly articles, so you are familiar with the structure, contents, and tone of research and quality improvement reports. You've critiqued research for assignments, so you know what a well-written research report requires. You have the foundational skills to do this—you just need a little guidance. This book will help you with that.

Navigating the publication process can be intimidating. Just choosing a journal to submit your work to from the hundreds of possibilities can seem daunting. Should you publish in an open access journal? And what exactly is that? How do you know if a journal is from one of those predatory publishers you've heard about? There are criteria and guidelines and forms to be filled out. There are ethical and legal considerations. And there's the online submission process to wade through.

This book is designed to guide you step-by-step through the process of rewriting your dissertation or DNP project paper into a high-quality manuscript ready to be submitted for publication and then guide you through the process of submitting it. It gives you the background information you need to confidently navigate the world of scholarly publishing.

Let's get started! It's time to become a published author!

1

THE BEGINNING

1

THE ESSENTIALS

This chapter discusses the difference between writing for school and writing for publication. It gives you a general overview of what needs to be done to go from a dissertation/scholarly project paper to a published article.

The first step to becoming an author is to start thinking of yourself as an author. You're no longer writing a paper—you're writing a *manuscript*. A manuscript is very different from a student paper. Although the purpose of your research or project hasn't changed, the purpose of your writing has. And so has your audience. You're no longer writing for professors who want evidence of your learning. Now you're writing for readers—clinicians, researchers, educators, policymakers—who want information they can *use*.

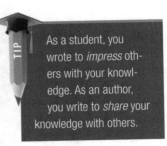

As a student, you wrote to *impress* others with your knowledge. As an author, you write to *share* your knowledge with others.

Student Paper vs. Manuscript: Purpose

The primary purpose of a student paper is to show the professor that you have an in-depth understanding of a topic and that you are able to communicate that understanding in a well-written scholarly paper. This is true even of your dissertation or project paper. A lot of the information is there to show your professors that all the decisions you made—from choosing your topic onward—were thoughtful and appropriate and grounded in the concepts and processes learned throughout your education.

The primary purpose of a manuscript isn't to demonstrate what *you* know; it's to share with readers what *they* need to know. Your first challenge as an author is figuring out what it is, among all that information your paper holds, that readers need to know. It is key to taking a 100- to 200-page dissertation or project paper and reshaping it into a 20- to 30-page manuscript.

Student Paper vs. Manuscript: Supporting Information

A lot of the supporting information in a student paper is there for the benefit of the professor. You "support" your decisions with evidence, expert opinion, and detailed descriptions of methodological choices. Supporting information is needed in a manuscript as well, just not as extensively. For example, you need to include the information about your methodology so that the reader can have confidence in your results or replicate the project, but not detailed explanations of all the methodological choices you made (unless those choices are unusual or open to debate).

Student Paper vs. Manuscript: Length

In a student paper, you kept writing until you had written at least as many pages as the professor required. Often that meant adding a little padding to get you there. Conciseness was not a virtue. That's not true for a manuscript. You will more often find yourself agonizing over what to delete to get your paper down to the word count the journal allows. It's a challenge to take dozens of pages of material—all of which you think is important or it wouldn't be there—and cut three-quarters of it. To do so, you have to consider every word that goes into a manuscript, which is exactly what a good writer should do.

By now, you've probably figured out that a key feature of revising your dissertation or project paper for publication is figuring out what information stays and what information goes. The chapters in Section 2 of this book, "Step-by-Step," will help you do that.

Essentials of Writing for Publication

It can feel daunting to face the prospect of turning your paper into a manuscript and figuring out how the publication process works.

It helps to know what to expect and what is expected of you before you get into the nitty gritty of rewriting your paper. Following are the essentials you need to know to get you started on your way to becoming an author.

Do Good Work

The number-one rule of writing for publication has nothing to do with writing. It's *do good work*. Good work starts with using a rigorous approach to address a significant issue. It contributes something important to the literature or practice.

Fatal flaws kill manuscripts. Fatal flaws are problems with research methodology or project planning and implementation that cannot be fixed after the fact. You can fill in gaps in your Literature Review or strengthen a weak Discussion, but no amount of revising is going to overcome poor methodology once a project is completed.

Remember how you learned to critique research articles way back when in your nursing program? You need to do that—with clear-eyed honesty—with your own work. Use the checklists at the end of this chapter to do a critical appraisal of your research methodology (there's one for qualitative and quantitative) or scholarly practice project.

Rewrite

One of the biggest mistakes people make when setting out to publish their dissertation or project is thinking of it as a revision. You need to approach the process as *rewriting* the paper versus *revising* it. If you just cut pieces and move things around, you will end up with a choppy, disorganized manuscript full of gaps and redundancies. Yes, there will be pieces and sections you can bring into the new manuscript, particularly from the Methods and Results sections. But you will have to do a lot of rewriting of the Introduction, Literature Review, and Discussion sections: combining, connecting, and resynthesizing the essential text into a coherent, integrated new whole.

Make It New

Regardless of what kind of manuscript you're writing, it has to add something new to the literature. Journals have limited pages, and journal editors are not going to waste them publishing information that is available elsewhere. It may be the findings of your study or the approach you took to address a systems problem. It could be establishing the state of the science in an integrative literature review or synthesizing the literature to determine evidence-based practice.

Follow Guidelines

Researchers have developed guidelines to standardize the reporting of research and health system change projects. The criteria in these guidelines are recognized as the standard for rigor and transparency in reporting research studies or quality improvement (QI) initiatives. The purpose is to ensure that scholarly work—particularly research and health system change projects—is reported accurately, clearly, and with transparency. Authors use these guidelines as they write up research and practice change reports, editors when they review manuscripts for publication, and readers when they must critically appraise articles for use in practice.

The International Committee of Medical Journal Editors (ICMJE) is a group of medical editors that meets yearly to determine best practice in conducting and reporting research. They produce standards— known as Recommendations for the Conduct, Reporting, Editing, and Publication of Scholarly Work in Medical Journals—that all credible peer-reviewed journals follow. The recommendations cover all aspects of scholarly publication for authors, editors, and publishers.

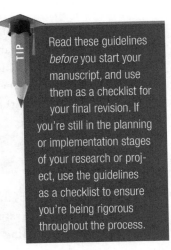

TIP

Read these guidelines *before* you start your manuscript, and use them as a checklist for your final revision. If you're still in the planning or implementation stages of your research or project, use the guidelines as a checklist to ensure you're being rigorous throughout the process.

Publication Standards and Guidelines

Research	ICMJE International Committee of Medical Journal Editors http://www.icmje.org/
Quality Improvement and Practice Change	SQUIRE Standards for Quality Improvement Reporting Excellence http://www.squire-statement.org/
Systematic Reviews	PRISMA Preferred Reporting Items for Systematic Reviews and Meta-Analyses http://www.prisma-statement.org/
Randomized Controlled Trials	CONSORT Consolidated Standards of Reporting Trials http://www.consort-statement.org/
Nonrandomized Studies	TREND Transparent Reporting of Evaluations with Nonrandomized Designs http://www.cdc.gov/trendstatement/

You will notice similarities among the various guidelines. That is because, regardless of whether you're doing research or practice change, certain components are essential. These include an introduction to the topic and its significance, background information so the reader understands the topic, consideration of ethical issues, rigorous methodology, information on what was evaluated and how, clearly delineated results, and a discussion of what everything means.

ICMJE established the Introduction, Methods, Results, and Discussion (IMRAD) structure that serves as the standard format for research and practice change articles.

> Introduction. This section introduces the topic and establishes significance. Included in this are the Background and Literature Review. You may decide to make each of these its own section with a corresponding subhead. The Introduction ends with a clear purpose statement. In a research article, the research questions may be included and, for quantitative studies, the hypotheses as well.

> Methods. The Methods sections in a research article detail the methodology of the study, including the sampling plan and data analysis. In a practice change article, you include the design of the project, the people involved in the project, and how outcomes are to be evaluated, including data collection.

> Results. The Results section of a research article is a straightforward account of the results of the data analysis without comments or interpretation. In a practice change article, this section becomes a little more complicated. Along with outcomes of the evaluation, you include a description of how the implementation process proceeded, any challenges that arose and how they were addressed, and unintended consequences.

Discussion. The Discussion section is where you tell the readers what everything means. You provide a summary of the key findings and put them into context with what is known from the literature. Study or project limitations are included in this section. The implications for research or practice are also incorporated; for a practice change, you address sustainability as well. A Conclusion also fits under this section, although it may have its own subheading.

Specific Guidelines

There are specific guidelines for different types of articles. These guidelines address the substance of your manuscript—ensuring that content is thorough, accurate, and presented in a clear, organized manner. Most scholarly journals will require manuscripts submitted to them follow the applicable guideline while also providing their own journal-specific requirements that address formatting, length, and structure.

SQUIRE

The SQUIRE guidelines provide a framework for reporting systems-level quality improvement (QI) and practice change projects. The framework uses the IMRAD structure; however, within each section are elements that differ from those in a research study.

PRISMA

The PRISMA guidelines provide a checklist of the 27 items you need to include in reporting a systematic review or meta-analysis. You should use these as a guide for integrative reviews as well, although all the items may not apply; for example, there aren't registered review protocols for integrative reviews. The PRISMA website also has a downloadable flow diagram template in a Word document format that's ready for you to plug in to your search strategy results.

CONSORT

The CONSORT guidelines are specifically for manuscripts reporting on randomized controlled trials (RCTs). Similar to PRISMA, CONSORT guidelines provide a detailed checklist of what information you need to include. The website also has a downloadable flow diagram for reporting the enrollment and progress of the study participants.

TREND

The TREND statement provides a 22-item checklist for use when reporting on nonrandomized controlled trials. It was developed for use specifically with intervention studies in behavioral and public health.

Journal Guidelines

Finally, there are the individual journal guidelines. Along with the publication standards and recommendations mentioned already, each journal has detailed author guidelines for manuscripts, including manuscript length, formatting, organization and headings, structure, and so on. Before starting

> **TIP**
>
> Don't try to contort your work to fit the guidelines. Consider each of the items in the guideline to determine if it's appropriate for your research or project. You also need to consider the author guidelines of the journal where you're submitting your work. But, at a minimum, you must include all the items showing that *your topic is significant, your methods were rigorous and ethical, and your outcomes are valid.*

your manuscript, read through the author guidelines for journals you're considering for submission so you know the page count and formatting that are required.

For a more detailed discussion of journal guidelines, see Chapter 9, "The Submission Process."

Formatting Styles

Most nursing journals use the American Psychological Association (APA) or the American Medical Association (AMA) formatting styles for the text and references. The biggest, although not the only, difference between the two is how references are cited in the text and reference list. APA cites the authors and year in the text and then lists them in alphabetical order in the reference list. AMA numbers the citations consecutively by order of appearance in the text and the reference list. There are other differences as well, so make sure you obtain the most up-to-date style manual for whatever formatting style is required.

	APA	AMA
In text	In a recent study of DNP projects, the researchers found that the majority of projects were staff education programs (Roush & Tesoro, 2018).	In a recent study of DNP projects, the researchers found that the majority of projects were staff education programs.[1]
In reference list	Roush, K., & Tesoro, M. (2018). An examination of the rigor and value of final scholarly projects completed by DNP nursing students. *Journal of Professional Nursing, 34*(6), 437–443.	1. Roush K, Tesoro M. An examination of the rigor and value of final scholarly projects completed by DNP nursing students. *Journal of Professional Nursing.* 2018;34(6):437–443.

Determine Authorship

What does it mean to be an author? Outside the world of scholarly publishing, we think of authors as people who write something themselves—every word of it. It's more complicated in scholarly publishing because often many people work on a project that eventually becomes a manuscript. Some people are involved in every aspect, from conceiving the idea to writing the final manuscript draft, as you were with your dissertation or project. Others may be involved only with pieces of it, such as statisticians who assist with data analysis or a committee member who gives feedback on your Literature Review.

All credible, scholarly journals follow the ICMJE criteria for authorship. To qualify as an author, you have to meet *all* the following criteria:

1. Substantial contributions to the conception or design of the work; or the acquisition, analysis, or interpretation of data for the work; AND

2. Drafting the work or revising it critically for important intellectual content; AND

3. Final approval of the version to be published; AND

4. Agreement to be accountable for all aspects of the work in ensuring that questions related to the accuracy or integrity of any part of the work are appropriately investigated and resolved.

(International Committee of Medical Journal Editors, 2019)

Members of your dissertation or project committee don't automatically qualify as authors on manuscripts. Usually your chairperson will because this person is closely involved in all phases of the research or project. However, that's not always the case with other committee members. For those who don't meet the criteria for authorship, you can recognize their contributions through an acknowledgement.

When there are multiple authors, one of them is designated as the corresponding author for the manuscript. All communication about the manuscript goes through this person. The corresponding author can be any of the authors; it doesn't have to be the first author. You are the corresponding author for manuscripts related to your dissertation or project. As the corresponding author, your contact information is published with the article, so give your professional, not your personal, email address.

For a more detailed discussion of authorship, see Chapter 7.

> **TIP**
>
> Conversations about authorship can be difficult—especially when it is a student–committee member relationship. There is still an expectation on the part of many faculty that they are automatically included on any publications related to their students' work. It may help to begin a conversation about the ICMJE criteria with your chairperson and ask for guidance as to where each committee member fits within that framework.

One more thought about authorship—how do you want your name to appear in the literature? If you start out using a middle initial, include it in your name for every article going forward. That's important as you build your recognition in your field. Also, keep in mind that if you have a hyphenated surname or spell out your middle name, it may lead to confusion in the indexing. For example, if you use Mary Kathryn Smith, there may be times you're indexed under Smith and others where you're indexed under Kathryn Smith.

What to Publish?

The major publication to come out of your doctoral work is the research or project report. Most of this book is about how to write that manuscript. However, a number of different manuscripts can come out of your work. Here are some of them.

Literature Review

When you rewrite your dissertation or project, you must whittle down your Literature Review to two or three pages. You'll have a lot of information left over that can be valuable to others. That leaves you with a wealth of information to turn into another manuscript. Systematic and integrative reviews have the best potential for publication because the systematic approach ensures that they are nonbiased and rigorous. However, many journals will publish a comprehensive literature review of a topic if it's put into a context that brings value to readers—that provides a synthesis of the literature that informs practice. See Chapter 4, "Methods and Analysis," for how to rewrite a Literature Review section for a research or project report and how to write a Literature Review as a manuscript.

Methods Paper

Was there an aspect of your methodology that was unique, particularly challenging, or innovative? Perhaps you had to overcome challenges with sampling or you used an unusual or rarely used statistical analysis method. If so, a methods paper may be in order. An innovative approach to recruiting a hard-to-reach population, strategies to overcome implementation barriers, and a critical discussion of ethical issues encountered in research with a vulnerable population are all examples of method topics that could be valuable for others.

Concept Analysis

A concept analysis is another possible manuscript. If you completed a formal concept analysis paper, it's one of the easier papers to turn into a manuscript because it starts out closer to what a first manuscript draft should be than other types of assignments. For it to be publishable, you need to make sure you've established the need for the analysis to be done, used a rigorous accepted method (such as

Rodgers or Walker & Avant), and presented a logical and valid analysis. For examples of clearly organized concept analyses, check out the ones published in the *Journal of Advanced Nursing*.

Application Paper

Translation of research to practice is one of the challenges in evidence-based healthcare. There's a continuing disconnect between the two, but writing an application paper is a great way to make that connection. You put your findings in the context of prior evidence and then show, *clearly and concretely*, how to apply them in a practice area. Depending on your topic, you can write a clinical application paper, a paper for nursing educators, or a policy paper. Sometimes you can write all three!

Example of Potential Manuscripts

Suppose you conducted your dissertation research on gender power related to maternal health. You needed to define the concept of gender power, conduct a comprehensive literature search and synthesize the results, and design and conduct the research. You have material for at least three manuscripts: a concept analysis of gender power, a literature review of gender power in maternal health, and the final research report.

ALERT!

No salami-slicing! That's when you try to slice one study or project into multiple papers that each have a limited amount of information or present the same information from a different angle. Every paper has to add genuinely unique and valuable information to the literature. For more information on this, see Chapter 7, "Ethics and Legalities."

Getting Started

Prioritize your writing. Set aside a time you'll spend writing, regardless of other obligations. It's too easy to let every other thing you have to do get in the way of sitting yourself down at the computer and facing that blank computer screen. Don't set yourself up to fail with an overly ambitious plan. Once you bypass your scheduled writing time, it gets easier to let it go by again. And again. Figure out what is realistically feasible for you, and then stick to it.

Set deadlines. Give yourself a schedule for getting sections of the manuscript written. If you're sending a query, you need to let the Editor-in-Chief know approximately when the manuscript will be ready for submission. Give yourself a reasonable amount of time to finish.

Check out your journal of choice. Journals vary in their requirements, format, and style, so knowing where you plan to submit before you start rewriting is helpful. Read the author guidelines of the journal you plan to submit to. Look at articles of the same type as yours and note how they're organized. You can use their organizational structure as a template for your article. Some journals have a set structure for research or QI articles that you're required to follow. Knowing that ahead of time will guide you in organizing your paper and save you from needing to revise down the road to meet author guidelines. Even if the journal is flexible with the structure, it helps to see how the articles are organized and get a sense of the tone of writing in accepted manuscripts. For example, are the Introduction, Background, and Literature Review sections divided under their own headings or combined in some way? How long are the sections? Do the articles include many tables and figures?

You can send a query before you start writing so that you know for sure where you're submitting your manuscript. For help with choosing a journal and sending a query, see Chapter 9.

Don't worry if you've already started or you change your selected journal. Once you have the main rewriting of the dissertation or project finished, you can add headings or reorganize the manuscript to meet the requirements of where you're submitting.

Step-By-Step

Getting Started

1. Consider what manuscripts you will write from your dissertation/ project paper.

2. Determine authorship and contact dissertation/project committee members as needed.

3. Prioritize your writing.

4. Create a writing schedule with deadlines.

5. Read through different journals that publish on your topic.

6. Read the author guidelines from two or three journals you're considering for submission.

7. Send a query to two or three journals (see Chapter 9).

8. Review the publication standards and guidelines for the type of manuscript you're writing.

9. Read Chapter 2, "Writing Well."

10. Start rewriting!

Self-Appraisal for Qualitative Methodology

❏ Does the study contribute useful new knowledge?

❏ Research Question and Purpose

- Is the research question clear?
- Is the purpose clearly stated?

❏ Theoretical Framework

- Did I identify a theoretical or conceptual framework?
- If not, does its absence detract from the study?
- Is the theoretical or conceptual framework appropriate for the research question?

❏ Study Design

- Does the design fit the question?

❏ Setting

- Is setting appropriate for the purpose and the population?

❏ Sample

- Did I adequately describe the sample selection procedures?
- Did I specify the inclusion and exclusion criteria?
- Was the sampling strategy appropriate?
- Did I achieve sampling saturation?

❏ Methodology

- Is data collection adequately described?
- Did I use the best method for collecting data?
- Did I use the appropriate data collection instrument?
- Was the instrument pretested?
- Did the interview questions adequately cover complexities of the phenomena?
- Was wording of interview questions clear and sensitive?
- Did I word the interview questions to avoid biased responses?

- ❏ Methodological Rigor
    - Did I use the appropriate techniques to ensure methodological rigor?
    - Did I establish trustworthiness?
    - Did I keep an audit trail?
    - Did I engage in reflexivity?
- ❏ Data Analysis
    - Were data analysis techniques appropriate?
    - Are coding schemes adequately described?
    - Is coding logical and complete?
    - Do themes appear to capture the meanings of the narratives?
    - Is analysis parsimonious?
- ❏ Limitations
    - Did I identify all relevant limitations?
- ❏ Ethical Aspects
    - Were measures taken to prevent harm and discomfort for participants?
    - Did data collection methods put any undue burden on the participants?
    - Was there any coercion or deception?
    - Did I obtain appropriate consent from all the participants?
    - Did I protect the privacy of participants?
    - If my population included vulnerable participants, did I have precautions in place to protect them?

(Gray, Grove, & Sutherland, 2017; Polit & Beck, 2017)

Self-Appraisal for Quantitative Methodology

❑ Does the study contribute useful new knowledge?

❑ Research Questions and Hypotheses

- Are the research questions clear?
- Are hypotheses based on theory or previous research?

❑ Theoretical Framework

- Did I identify a theoretical framework?
- Is the theoretical framework appropriate for the research question?

❑ Study Design

- Does the design fit the question?
- Did I adequately describe any interventions?
- If there was an intervention, did I use an appropriate experimental or quasi-observational design?
- Was the time dimension (cross-sectional, longitudinal) appropriate?

❑ Setting

- Is the setting appropriate for the purpose and the population?

❑ Sample

- Did I clearly delineate inclusion and exclusion criteria?
- Is the sampling strategy appropriate?
- Did I use a recruitment strategy that avoided sampling bias?
- Did the sampling strategy yield a representative sample?
- Did I do a power analysis to determine the appropriate sample size?
- Did I end up with an adequate sample size?

- ❑ Methodology
  - Is data collection adequately described?
  - Did I use the best method for collecting data?
  - Did I report psychometrics for data collection instruments?
  - Did I establish reliability of the instruments for my study population?
- ❑ Data Analysis
  - Were correct descriptive statistics used?
  - Did I meet assumptions for inferential statistics?
  - Did I use the appropriate statistical tests for the level of measurement of variables?
  - Were correct statistical tests used for any multivariate procedures?
- ❑ Limitations
  - Did I identify all relevant limitations?
- ❑ Ethical Aspects
  - Were measures taken to prevent harm and discomfort for participants?
  - Did data collection methods put any undue burden on the participants?
  - Was there any coercion or deception?
  - Did I obtain appropriate consent from all the participants?
  - Did I protect the privacy of participants?
  - If my population included vulnerable participants; did I have precautions in place to protect them?

(Gray, Grove, & Sutherland, 2017; Polit & Beck, 2017)

Resources

American Psychological Association. (2010). *Publication manual* (6th ed.). Washington, DC: Author.

Des Jarlais, D. C., Lyles, C., Crepaz, N., & TREND Group. (2004). Improving the reporting quality of nonrandomized evaluations of behavioral and public health interventions: The TREND statement. *American Journal of Public Health, 94*(3), 361–366.

Gray, J. R., Grove, S. K., & Sutherland, S. (2017). *Burns and Grove's The practice of nursing research: Appraisal, synthesis, and generation of evidence* (8th ed.). St Louis, MO: Elsevier Health Sciences.

Moher, D., Liberati, A., Tetzlaff, J., & Altman, D. G. (2010). Preferred reporting items for systematic reviews and meta-analyses: The PRISMA statement. *International Journal of Surgery, 8*(5), 336–341.

Ogrinc, G., Davies, L., Goodman, D., Batalden, P., Davidoff, F., & Stevens, D. (2015). SQUIRE 2.0 (standards for quality improvement reporting excellence): Revised publication guidelines from a detailed consensus process. *The Journal of Continuing Education in Nursing, 46*(11), 501–507.

Polit, D. F., & Beck, C. T. (2017). *Nursing research: Generating and assessing evidence for nursing practice* (10th ed.). Philadelphia, PA: Lippincott Williams & Wilkins.

Rodgers, B. (2000). Concept analysis: An evolutionary view. In B. Rodgers & K. Knafl, *Concept development in nursing: Foundations, techniques and applications* (2nd ed., pp. 77–101). Philadelphia, PA: W. B. Saunders.

Roush, K., & Tesoro, M. (2018). An examination of the rigor and value of final scholarly projects completed by DNP nursing students. *Journal of Professional Nursing, 34*(6), 437–443.

Schulz, K. F., Altman, D. G., & Moher, D. (2010). CONSORT 2010 statement: Updated guidelines for reporting parallel group randomised trials. *BMC Medicine, 8*(1), 18.

Walker, L. O., & Avant, K. C. (2018). *Strategies for theory construction in nursing* (6th ed.). Chicago, IL: Pearson.

Reference

International Committee of Medical Journal Editors. (2019). *Recommendations for the conduct, reporting, editing, and publication of scholarly work in medical journals.* Retrieved from http://www.icmje.org/

2

WRITING WELL

Academic writing has the reputation of being tedious to read, but yours doesn't have to be that way. You're writing about something you care about; don't leave it lying there flat and lifeless on the page. Good scholarly writing is engaging, informative, accurate, and clear. Write with authority and energy. This chapter will help you do that.

Clarity Is Key!

The most important characteristic of good scholarly writing is clarity—you want the reader to understand the information exactly as you intend it to be understood. You accomplish that through careful use of language, adhering to proper sentence structure, and providing specific details.

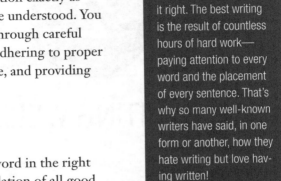

TIP

Don't be discouraged if you find writing difficult and time-consuming. That just means you're doing it right. The best writing is the result of countless hours of hard work—paying attention to every word and the placement of every sentence. That's why so many well-known writers have said, in one form or another, how they hate writing but love having written!

Language

Using the right word in the right place is the foundation of all good writing. Every word you choose should be the best possible word to convey the information you want to share. This is true for all writing, whether you're writing poetry or a novel or a research report. However, there are certain pitfalls that scholarly writers are particularly prone to, such as the use of "academese" or jargon. Learning to use language that is energized, clear, and precise will go a long way toward completing a manuscript that is engaging for the reader and valuable to the science.

Use Straightforward Language

Don't try to sound smart. Remember, your goal isn't to impress readers with your intelligence; it's to share information. Presenting complex information in easily understood, everyday language is the best way to do that. Using straightforward language doesn't mean "dumbing down" the information. It also doesn't mean avoiding all technical terms. You should use sophisticated or technical language when the material calls for it. Using straightforward language does mean choosing words for clarity and conciseness rather than for effect.

Look up the definition of any word that you don't use regularly or have the slightest question about its meaning. With online dictionaries, it takes only a minute.

Straightforward language is more concise—giving you more space for meaningful information. Often, one word can replace a phrase. See the examples in this table.

Overly Complicated	Straightforward
Take into consideration	Consider
In the event that	If
Be of the opinion	Think, believe, feel
With the exception of	Except
For the purpose of	For, to
By means of	By
At the present time	Now, currently
In a situation in which	When
In view of the fact	Because, as
A large majority of	Most
Has the capacity of	Can
Are in agreement	Agree
In excess of	More than

Here are a few examples of the difference using straightforward language can make with clarity and conciseness.

Overly Complicated	Simple and Easy-to-Understand
Staff education involved providing NICU nurses with didactic and written education to facilitate their comprehension of the intervention.	We provided the NICU nurses with classes and handouts so they would understand the intervention.
Subsequent to commencing the intervention, we procured two weeks of discharge data.	After starting the intervention, we collected two weeks of discharge data.
Findings were positive for the presence of lower rates of readmissions in the intervention group.	There were lower rates of readmissions in the intervention group.

No Jargon, Colloquialisms, or Euphemisms

Use language that will be understood accurately by anyone reading the paper, including those outside of healthcare professions or living in different regions of the country. Readers can easily misinterpret jargon, colloquialisms, and euphemisms.

Jargon

Jargon is specialized language used by a group, such as nurses and other healthcare providers. We use it so routinely that it can slip into our writing unnoticed. The following table lists some common jargon examples.

Jargon	Correct Terminology
Bagged	Ventilated with a bag-valve-mask
Call a code	Call the cardiopulmonary resuscitation team
Crash cart	Emergency cart or resuscitation cart
Drop a tube	Insert a nasogastric tube

IV push	Administer medications via IV
Pass meds	Administer medications
Run fluids	Administer intravenous fluids

Medical abbreviations and technical terms are not considered jargon in a scholarly manuscript. Don't use medical abbreviations that are short for Latin terms, such as prn and ad lib, in the text. However, you can use abbreviations for other medical phrases, such as range of motion (ROM), anterior cruciate ligament (ACL), or red blood cells (RBCs) after first writing them out in the text.

Colloquialisms

Colloquialisms are informal words or phrases that may be figurative (also called an idiom) or associated with a specific geographic region. They are never appropriate in a scholarly manuscript.

Following are examples of colloquialisms:

- Do the heavy lifting
- Open a can of worms
- Just the bare bones
- Tough nut to crack
- Turn for the worse
- Fell through the cracks
- Wade through
- Digging deeper
- Right off the bat

Euphemisms

Euphemisms are words you use when you want to soften a difficult or harsh statement. One of the common uses is when talking about death. People say *passed away* instead of *died*; or they say *put to sleep* when talking about euthanizing a pet. Although commonly used in conversation, euphemisms are not appropriate in scholarly manuscripts.

Concision

Every word that doesn't add to a reader's understanding detracts from it. Your job is to present information with the fewest, most precise words possible so that readers don't have to wade through a cluttered manuscript to figure out what to pay attention to.

> *"Mozart: There are just as many notes, Majesty, as are required. Neither more nor less."*
>
> *From* Amadeus *screenplay*

An added benefit to writing concisely is that it gives you more room for all the important stuff as you try to whittle down your dissertation or project paper.

Start by getting rid of meaningless words and phrases. For example, do you need to begin a sentence with *it goes without saying*? If it goes without saying, why are you saying it?

Check your manuscript for any of the following words and phrases. Delete them and see what happens. In most cases you won't miss them, and you will end up with a sharpened focus on the actual information.

- Actually
- Truly

- Really

- Basically

- Obviously

- Practically

- In terms of _____

- It goes without saying _____

- In the area of _____

- It is necessary to _____

- All in all _____

- In order to _____

- All things considered _____

Take a look at this example of the difference that getting rid of meaningless words and phrases can make. The resulting sentence is more focused and energized after half the words were removed without any loss of meaning.

Before:
It is important to note that when actually implementing the intervention, the nurses will obviously not have access to the concealed answers.

After:
The nurses will not have access to the answers during implementation.

While you're removing meaningless words and phrases, delete any adjectives, adverbs, qualifiers, and intensifiers as well. Then read through and see if any of them need to be replaced for an objective, accurate understanding of the material.

Examples of qualifiers:

- Basically
- May/Might
- Probably/Possibly
- Seems/Appears
- Somewhat
- Sort of
- Some/Most/Many/Few
- Sometimes/Usually
- Mostly

Examples of intensifiers:

- A lot
- Ever
- Quite
- Really
- So
- Too
- Very

If you do think an adverb is needed, try to replace it with a strong verb.

Examples of adverb replacements are shown in this table.

Cried uncontrollably	Sobbed
Ate quickly	Devoured
Held tightly	Grasped
Reached clumsily	Fumbled
Quickly moved forward	Lunged
Desperately try	Strive or struggle

Do the same for intensifiers as well, particularly *very*. For example, *very hungry* becomes *ravenous*, *very thin* becomes *cachectic*, and *very painful* becomes *agonizing*.

Qualifiers, such as *somewhat*, *seems*, or *some*, make your statements sound tentative, so use them judiciously. In research findings, absolutisms are not warranted, and words such as *indicates* or *suggests* are appropriate.

Active Voice

Use active voice. With active voice, the subject acts upon the object instead of the object being acted upon. Active voice brings energy and clarity and is more concise. It also makes it clear who or what the subject is in the sentence. This is important for clarity. Take a look at the difference in the following examples.

Passive Voice	Active Voice
Gastric emptying is inhibited by cholecystokinin, which also sends satiety signals to the hypothalamus via the vagal nerve.	Cholecystokinin inhibits gastric emptying and sends satiety signals to the hypothalamus via the vagal nerve.
The participants were instructed by the physical therapist on how to use the equipment before they began the protocol.	The physical therapist instructed the participants on how to use the equipment before they began the protocol.

Personal Pronouns

Using personal pronouns is OK and actually preferred. Referring to yourself in the third person sounds pretentious and makes for awkward sentences. Trying to avoid saying *I* or *We* increases use of the passive voice. Look at the difference in the following.

Avoiding a personal pronoun:

- This researcher recruited participants at community health fairs.

- Participants were recruited at community health fairs.

Using a personal pronoun:

- I recruited participants at community health fairs.

The first example sounds pretentious, and in the second, the reader doesn't know who did the recruiting. The third sounds more natural and clearly identifies who did the recruiting.

Be Precise

Be precise, and choose your words carefully. Make sure your words are communicating exactly what you intend they communicate. Many words have connotations that affect their literal meaning in positive or negative ways. For example, consider the word *selective*. It means to choose carefully. *Discerning* and *picky* are also words that mean to choose carefully, but they have different connotations than the more neutral *selective*.

In scientific writing, you should also avoid using statistical terms for nonstatistical use. These terms include *significant, normal, random, correlate,* and *sample*.

Use concrete nouns. A concrete noun is tangible—it represents something you can see, smell, touch, or taste. When you use a concrete noun, you have control over the image created in a reader's mind. The image will be similar, if not identical, for everyone. That's not so for an abstract noun. When you use abstract terms, such as love, cour-age, caring, or health, readers interpret them through their own lens. That leaves room for different interpretations, which may or may not be what you intended.

> **TIP**
>
> The thesaurus is a great tool, but use it carefully. Do not insert words indiscriminately. That is where you can get in trouble with different connotations among words with similar meanings.

Redundancy

Watch for redundancy. Repetition slips into your writing in differ-ent ways. Most often it's unconscious—using common redundant phrases, for instance. Sometimes it's purposeful for emphasis or to make sure the reader will understand what you're trying to say. Don't be redundant. Redundancy kills clarity and conciseness and wastes precious space.

Do not repeat statements for emphasis. Do not reword the same information. It will not enhance a reader's understanding of the material. Say your idea clearly using straightforward language the first and only time. If you think a reader will need help under-standing something, it's better to use examples than to repeat the information using different words.

People use hundreds of redundant phrases without realizing it. Following is a list of some of them. Stay alert to these and others in your manuscript.

Examples of redundant phrases:

- Difficult dilemma
- Absolutely necessary
- 12 noon or 12 midnight
- Different varieties
- New innovation
- Entirely eliminate
- Past history
- Hopefully optimistic
- Revert back
- The reason is because
- Advance preview
- Compete with each other
- Descend down
- Face mask
- First conceived
- Join together
- Plunge down

Do not cover the same information in multiple places. If you've covered information or talked about studies in the Introduction, do not repeat it in the Discussion. You can refer back to material if you're adding something new—such as putting it in the context of your research findings or building on it for application to practice. Information in multiple places is often a sign of a poorly organized paper. See the "Organization" section coming up for help on establishing a logical flow of information in your manuscript.

Specificity

Vague general statements dilute the value of your paper. Generalities do not add to a reader's understanding; instead, they leave room for misinterpretation. You can start with a general statement, but you need to then provide specific details. For example, if you say that staff turnover is a barrier to quality care, you have to then say why and how. You don't need to write a lot about it; you can give details for context in a sentence or two. Use concrete nouns, as described earlier. Using examples is an excellent way to add specificity and enhance a reader's understanding.

Organization

A well-organized manuscript takes the reader smoothly from the first page to the last without detours or reruns. You accomplish this by establishing a logical flow of information, avoiding redundancy, and using subheads and transitional devices.

Logical Flow

Keep in mind that you have all the connections in your head, but the readers don't; you have to make those connections clear for them. You have to introduce an idea before talking about it. You can't tell readers how to implement the three available strategies for a problem without having first told them that there are three available strategies.

The standard advice is to present information from the general to the specific. This usually works, but there are times you may want to start with the specific and then move out to the general. It's important that the reader knows right away what the paper is about. If you're focusing in tightly on a topic, it's a good idea to start with that tight focus before pulling back to give background context. For example, if you're writing about stress incontinence, if you go from the general to the specific, you would start with incontinence in general and then focus on stress incontinence. But it could take a paragraph or two before the reader knows that the topic is specifically stress incontinence. Starting with specifics situates the reader right away.

Paragraphs

Each paragraph should have one main idea. Start with a topic sentence that clearly expresses that idea, and then build on it through explication using description, analysis, interpretation, and examples. Decide on an ordering scheme, whether it be chronological, cause and effect, importance, classification, or process, and be consistent with that order throughout the paragraph. Each sentence should flow logically into the next.

Checklist for organization:

❑ Each paragraph has one main idea.

❑ Each concept is introduced before it's talked about.

❑ The connection between the purpose and each idea, concept, and proposition is clear.

❑ Ideas introduced early in the manuscript are threaded through to the end.

Use Subheads

Subheads are a great way to cleanly organize your manuscript and keep the reader situated. They can serve as a transitional tool as well. Even if you don't plan on including subheads in your finished manuscript, subheads can help you get organized. You can delete them once you establish a good flow. Just make sure you transition the reader from one idea to the next.

Use Transitional Devices

You need to prepare the reader each time you move from one idea to another. You do this with transitional words, phrases, and statements. When you're shifting focus between paragraphs, you can use a transitional word or use the first sentence of the paragraph to summarize what the prior paragraph said, preparing the reader for what's coming next.

Take a look at how the italicized first sentence of the second paragraph below does this. The first paragraph covers health disparities in low- and middle-income countries and secondary to violence [*Health disparities are not only evident in differences between low- and high-income nations or in populations exposed to violent conflicts*], and the second paragraph shifts to talking about health disparities in high-income countries [*they also exist within high-income countries*].

Example of transitional statement:

> *Social, political, and economic factors affect health and well-being in profound and tangible ways throughout the world. In 2004, the life expectancy in low- and middle-income countries in Africa was only 49.2 years compared to that of 79.4 years in high-income countries in North America and Europe (World Health Organization, 2004). Ninety-nine percent of all deaths in children younger than 15 years and 83% of deaths in people 15 to 59 years are in the developing world. War and violence account for almost half of deaths in the latter group in the regions of sub-Saharan Africa, Latin America, and the Caribbean.*

> *Health disparities are not only evident in differences between low- and high-income nations or in populations exposed to violent conflicts, they also exist within high-income countries. In the United States, there are significant differences in health outcomes among socioeconomic, racial, and ethnic groups. For ex-*

ample, the infant mortality rate for African Americans, Native Americans, and Alaskan Natives is about twice that of White Americans. Socioeconomic differences in infant mortality have been found in Finland, Denmark, and Norway as well.

Transitional devices also establish relationships between ideas. They provide the reader with information about how to think about the connections between ideas.

ALERT!

Be careful in your choice of transitional words and phrases. Make sure you're picking the right one for the job it needs to do.

Transitional Words and Phrases

To Compare
- Similarly
- Likewise
- In the same way

To Contrast
- Yet
- However
- Though
- But
- In contrast

To Indicate Time
- While
- After
- Following
- Subsequently

To Show Addition
- Furthermore
- Additionally
- Finally
- Also
- In addition

To Show Effect
- Therefore
- Consequently
- Accordingly
- As a result
- Because

Regardless of what kind of paper you're writing, you're telling a story. There has to be a narrative flow. It's not just a series of sentences, one after the other. You create coherence and meaning by making sure each sentence has some connection to the one before and the one after. When you do that well, you can go to the last few sentences in your paper and clearly see their connection to the first few sentences. If the connection isn't obvious, you lost one or more of the narrative threads along the way.

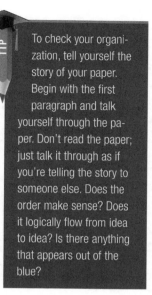

TIP

To check your organization, tell yourself the story of your paper. Begin with the first paragraph and talk yourself through the paper. Don't read the paper; just talk it through as if you're telling the story to someone else. Does the order make sense? Does it logically flow from idea to idea? Is there anything that appears out of the blue?

Grammar and Punctuation

Correct grammar is clear cut, with rules to follow. You can find dozens of resources to help you with grammar.

Grammar Resources

Grammarly
https://www.grammarly.com/blog/category/handbook/

Grammar Book
https://www.grammarbook.com

Grammar Girl
http://www.quickanddirtytips.com/grammar-girl

Purdue OWL Online Writing Lab
https://owl.purdue.edu/owl/purdue_owl.html

Final Steps

Review your manuscript on paper. Print your manuscript and read it on paper with a pen in hand. **Revise.**

Read your manuscript out loud. When you read your manuscript out loud, you will notice where you trip over awkward phrasing. Hearing it will also help you pick up on redundancies or missing information or when something is out of order. **Revise.**

Get feedback. Never send out a manuscript without getting feedback. People are never good reviewers of their own manuscript. It's easy to read what you think you wrote instead of what you actually wrote. You have all the information, so you don't notice gaps in thinking or missing connections.

Have two people read the manuscript: one person who knows the content and can give you feedback on accuracy and completeness of the information, and one person who doesn't know anything about the content and can let you know if the information is clearly presented and understandable. **Revise.**

Sleep on it. Once you get feedback and do your final revisions, put the manuscript away for a couple of days. Then do one more read, and if all is in good shape, submit!

Save each revision with a different filename. Keep it simple. Some people save each revision with the date. I prefer to use the alphabet because I tend to save multiple versions in a day. I start by saving the first revision with an A added to the end of the title and go on from there.

> TIP
>
> It's difficult to send your work out there to be judged. Revision is crucial, but at some point you have to *let go*. You'll get feedback from reviewers for any remaining revisions you need.

Step-By-Step

Odds and Ends

1. Never say *I believe*, *I think*, or *My opinion is...*

2. When referring to a medical doctor, use the term *physician*, not *doctor*.

3. Put the most important information at the beginning or at the end of a sentence or paragraph—those are the positions with the most power. Don't bury it in the middle.

4. Use the same term for a concept throughout the paper. An example is *organization* vs. *institution* vs. *facility*. Pick one and stick with it so you don't confuse the reader.

5. Be consistent with tense and point of view.

6. Consider whether statements that are general knowledge are needed. For example: *The population is aging. Healthcare is costly. Obesity is prevalent in the US.*

7. Use sentences of varying length throughout the paper.

8. Exclamation points have no place in scholarly writing.

9. Proofread your manuscript. Spelling and grammar programs are not infallible and won't pick up the words that are spelled correctly but are the wrong word. This happens often with words where only one letter differs, such as *if* and *of* or *meet* and *meat*.

Resources

American Psychological Association. (2010). *Publication manual* (6th ed.). Washington, DC: Author.

Dexter, P. (2000). Tips for scholarly writing in nursing. *Journal of Professional Nursing*, *16*(1), 6–12.

Strunk, W., and White, E. B. (2007). *The elements of style*. New York, NY: Penguin.

Zinsser, W. (2006). *On writing well* (7th ed.). New York, NY: Harper Perennial.

SECTION

2

STEP-BY-STEP

3

INTRODUCTION AND LITERATURE REVIEW

A well-written Introduction and Literature Review provide readers with all the information they need—and only the information they need—to understand the topic or problem, appreciate its significance, and see the need for doing the research or project. There cannot be any extraneous information, no matter how interesting it may be.

The Introduction takes on added importance in a manuscript because it's where you will either capture or lose readers' interest. If you don't convince them of the importance of the topic and the need for your research or project at the beginning, it's unlikely that they will continue reading. This is true also for the editor and reviewers who will decide if your manuscript is worthy of publication.

The first sentence of your manuscript needs to engage the reader. It should be a compelling statement that situates readers exactly where you want them to be. One caveat—the evidence has to be strong enough to support such a statement.

Look at the difference between two possible sentences for the beginning of a paper on the health effects of discrimination in LGBT individuals:

> *It appears that in many places in the United States, individuals may still face discrimination due to their sexual orientation and gender that can leave them feeling marginalized.*[1]

> *Lesbian, gay, bisexual, and transgender (LGBT) individuals continue to face significant discrimination and marginalization in the United States.*[1]

The first is wordy and full of qualifiers (appears, may, can) that make the author sound unsure and drain the statement of its power. The second presents the same information but with more confidence while also being more concise. (For more information on avoiding qualifiers in your writing, see Chapter 2, "Writing Well.")

Ideally, readers should know the focus of the manuscript within the first few sentences, but certainly within the first paragraph. Take a look at the following examples of the first sentences of research and quality improvement articles from the literature. Note how much information is contained within two sentences. And not just any information—each sentence provides the reader with information critical to understanding the subject and its importance. Also note how the authors introduce the *specific* subject of the paper (the underlined segments) right away, not just the general topic area. The title of the article precedes it.

CULTIVATING QUALITY: AN EVIDENCE-BASED PROTOCOL FOR MANAGING HYPOGLYCEMIA

Increased attention has been placed on <u>glycemic management</u> in the United States in response to the rising prevalence of diabetes and its associated economic burden (McEuen et al., 2010).

CULTIVATING QUALITY: REDUCING SURGICAL SITE INFECTIONS IN CHILDREN UNDERGOING CARDIAC SURGERY

Health care–associated infections in hospitalized patients are a significant cause of illness and result in an estimated 99,000 deaths annually. <u>Surgical site infections</u> (SSIs) account for one in five of all health care–associated infections and can lead to reoperation, longer hospitalization, and increased costs (Galvin, 2009).

CHILDREN'S COPING STRATEGIES FOR CHEMOTHERAPY-INDUCED NAUSEA AND VOMITING

<u>Pediatric</u> cancer treatment often includes the use of chemotherapy agents that can cause multiple and sometimes severe side effects. <u>Chemotherapy-induced nausea and vomiting</u> (CINV) is a common occurrence, with as many as 60% of pediatric patients with cancer reporting nausea or vomiting at some point during chemotherapy treatment (Rodgers et al., 2012).

STAFF NURSES' PERCEPTIONS REGARDING PALLIATIVE CARE FOR HOSPITALIZED OLDER ADULTS

For many <u>hospitalized older adults</u> with serious illnesses, early implementation of <u>palliative care</u> can be of critical importance. Many older patients have multiple chronic comorbidities, and may experience exacerbations that result in increased debility and alter their life circumstances (O'Shea, 2014).

COMMUNICATION AND OUTCOMES OF VISITS BETWEEN OLDER PATIENTS AND NURSE PRACTITIONERS

<u>Effective patient-clinician</u> communication is at the heart of good healthcare and may be <u>even more vital for older patients and their nurse practitioners</u> (NPs). The complex healthcare needs created by chronic illnesses and medication regimens of many older people require a greater exchange of information to achieve desired health outcomes (Gilbert & Hayes, 2009).

GIVING SEXUAL ASSAULT SURVIVORS TIME TO DECIDE: AN EXPLORATION OF THE USE AND EFFECTS OF THE NONREPORT OPTION

Forensic nurses, sexual assault nurse examiners (SANEs), and victim advocates have long recognized the trauma of sexual assault crimes and the <u>significance of survivors' decisions around reporting these crimes</u> to law enforcement agencies (Heffron, Busch-Armendariz, Vohra, Johnson, & Camp, 2014).

Let's take a look at what can happen when you don't start with the specific topic of your paper. Read the following two possible first sentences of an Introduction for a manuscript.

> *According to AACN (2018), a shortage of nurses is expected between now and 2030 due to the retirement of a large contingent of baby boomers along with increased demands for healthcare. This is further exacerbated by nursing programs having to turn away qualified applicants due to a lack of nursing faculty.*

What do you think is the focus of this paper? A developing nursing shortage? What about if we start off like this:

> *Making the move from clinical practice to academia is a challenging transition for new doctoral graduates. Not only do they face going from being an expert to a novice, they also must*

adjust to academic culture, learn new systems, develop and teach multiple new courses, get their research program off the ground, publish their dissertations, meet the needs of students, and acquire pedagogical skills.

Now what do you think is the focus of this paper? It's obvious that it's the transition of new doctoral graduates from clinical practice to academia. The first version starts with background information *related* to the topic, but the reader thinks it *is* the topic. It's not that that information doesn't belong in the paper; it's part of the significance. It just doesn't belong where it is, misleading the reader for the first paragraph.

Rewriting

ALERT!

Before you start rewriting the Introduction and Literature Review sections, go back to the literature and see if there is any new research that needs to be incorporated into your manuscript. Peer reviewers will note if you're missing an important recent study that has implications for your work.

Look at similar articles in the journal you're submitting to for guidance on how to organize the Introduction and Literature Review sections of your manuscript. There may be a set structure. For example, all the articles have a short Introduction followed by a more in-depth Literature Review section, or they have only an Introduction. In some articles, the Literature Review is identified as Background. We call it Literature Review in this chapter, but the structure and length of each section may vary even among the same types of articles, depending on what is needed for a particular paper. Some articles may combine the sections into one, whereas others separate them into distinct sections. The organization of your manuscript also depends on the type and the amount of information needed for a reader to understand the topic and appreciate its significance. In some cases, you may need only a short Introduction—perhaps because it's a well-known topic—whereas in other Introductions more information may be needed to provide sufficient descriptions about a complex group of variables or necessary contextual elements.

Regardless of the length and structure of the Introduction and Literature Review sections, the questions in Table 3.1 must be answered by the time you get to the end of your Introduction and Literature Review sections.

TABLE 3.1 Questions for Better Introduction and Literature Review Sections

What is happening?	Describe the topic or problem.
Why should we care?	Establish significance of the topic. Include only the most important prevalence and incidence statistics. Spend only one or two sentences on morbidity and mortality rates.
What is currently known or being done?	Provide an overview of the current state of the knowledge on your topic or prior efforts to address your problem. Support with evidence. Explicate with specifics from a few key studies.
What do we need to learn or do now, and why?	This is your purpose statement, PICO or research questions, or hypotheses. The justification for your purpose should be clear from your answers to the previous questions. If not, clarify why your questions, hypotheses, or approach are the logical thing to do or the best next step.

These are the same questions you answered in the Introduction and Literature Review sections of your dissertation or project paper. Just as you did in that paper, your answers should lead the reader logically and inevitably to your purpose statement or research questions. The difference in a manuscript is that you need to get there a lot quicker.

To do that, follow these three principles—*focus, discriminate, support.*

Focus. *Stay tightly focused on your purpose. The purpose statement drives everything and is the final determinant of what stays and what goes.*

Discriminate. *Include what allows you to be the most concise without losing key information.*

Support. *Determine which studies, among the many covered in your Literature Review, best support your ideas, actions, and conclusions.*

TIP

The purpose statement is the most important statement in your manuscript because it guides everything you write. Print it out in large font and keep it in view at all times. Make sure every sentence you write directly relates to the purpose and adds something unique to the reader's understanding of it.

You can further highlight the value of your study or project by stating outright how the results will be beneficial. A clear value statement tells the reader: *If we learn this or do this, then this positive thing could happen.* Such a statement should come just before or after your purpose statement. Following are some examples:

> *As such, understanding factors that exacerbate or attenuate bullying is important as they can lead to personalized efforts to prevent such behavior or be incorporated into schoolwide interventions* (Stoddard, Varela, & Zimmerman, 2015, p. 422).

> *Understanding the experiences of these women is crucial to provide effective interventions, strategies, and services to address the specific challenges they face. Therefore, we conducted a qualitative descriptive study to explore the lived experience of IPV for women in rural settings* (Roush & Kurth, 2016, p. 309).

Therefore, we conducted a study that examined the rigor and value of final practice projects completed by recent DNP graduates. Evaluating the rigor and value of these projects will help determine if DNP programs are producing nurses prepared to improve patient outcomes, influence healthcare policy, or make system changes that improve health care outcomes (Roush & Tesoro, 2018, p. 438).

Be systematic in your approach. Do not just start cutting and pasting from your dissertation or project paper. You will end up with a disorganized paper that has gaps and redundancy. Start by reading through the Introduction and Literature Review of your dissertation or project paper. Then write a brief summary answer to the questions in Table 3.1. Use that to guide your rewrite.

In your dissertation/project paper, there was overlap of information in your Introduction and Literature Review in answering the questions in Table 3.1. You need to eliminate that redundancy in the manuscript.

ALERT!

For a DNP quality improvement project, the purpose is what you hope to accomplish, not what you're going to do. If you're trying to lower the rates of pressure ulcers on your unit by forming a unit-based pressure ulcer prevention team, the purpose of the project is to lower the rate of pressure ulcers, not to form a unit-based pressure ulcer prevention team.

WRITE THIS: The purpose of this project was to lower the rate of pressure ulcers on the neurosurgery unit through the establishment of a unit-based pressure ulcer prevention team.

NOT THIS: The purpose of this project was to establish a neurosurgery unit-based pressure ulcer prevention team to lower the rate of pressure ulcers. (Written this way, if you've established the team, you've met the purpose, even if pressure ulcer rates don't decrease.)

In a practice project, you will have specific aims and objectives. You can include these as a bulleted list. For example, for the pressure ulcer project just discussed:

> *The purpose of this project was to lower the rate of pressure ulcers on the neurosurgery unit through the establishment of a unit-based pressure ulcer prevention team. The specific objectives were*
>
> > *(1) to decrease the rate of new pressure ulcers to less than 4% within one month of implementing the team*
> >
> > *(2) to decrease the rate to less than 2% after three months and sustain that rate over time.*

Quality Improvement and Evidence-Based Projects: Where to Fit the Local Problem

In some ways, a quality improvement (QI) manuscript is more difficult to organize because there are more moving parts. Along with the standard information included in the Introduction and Literature Review sections, you have to provide information specific to the problem in your setting.

It helps to create an outline and determine where information belongs before you start rewriting. That will help you avoid redundancy, which slips in easily in papers with complex organizational elements.

- Introduction to the topic and information to establish significance (What is happening, and why should we care?)

- Background that includes information about what is known about the problem in general (What is currently known or being done?)

- Local problem and background (What is happening specifically in your setting?)

- Literature review that supports your approach (What is currently known or being done?)

- Purpose and approach (What do we need to learn or do now?)

Again, include only the information readers need to understand what is happening, why it's a problem, and why you chose the approach you did.

TIP

In the Introduction and Literature Review sections, only include information you had before you started planning and implementing your study or project.

Getting to a First Draft

You can use the Introduction of your dissertation/project paper as a way into the first draft of the Introduction and Literature Review sections of your manuscript. In writing the Introduction of your dissertation or project paper, you provided a summary of what is currently known with little or no explication of specific studies. For the manuscript, you will need to tighten it considerably while also adding some details about specific studies from your Literature Review section.

Start by pulling out the topic sentence of each paragraph in your Introduction. Determine if any of these can be eliminated or combined while still answering the four questions in Table 3.1.

For example, in my dissertation on intimate partner violence in the rural setting, the Introduction was six pages long, with the following topic sentences at the beginning of each paragraph:

- Intimate partner violence (IPV) against women is a pervasive health and social problem in the United States.

- Intimate partner violence has serious short- and long-term negative physical and mental health consequences, including trauma, chronic pain, gastrointestinal disorders, gynecological problems, anxiety and mood disorders, substance abuse, and post-traumatic stress disorder (PTSD), and it results in impaired quality of life.

- IPV has significant economic costs as well.

- IPV presents unique challenges to women living in rural areas that increase their vulnerability, limit their options for seeking safety, and hamper efforts to leave an abusive relationship.

- In addition to difficulty obtaining protective services, studies consistently find that rural women face limited availability and access to resources, including emergency department resources, mental health services, and shelters.

- Another factor that causes increased difficulties for women in rural areas is geographical isolation.

- Sociocultural factors also increase vulnerability for women in the rural setting.

- Despite the evidence that women in the rural setting face a unique set of challenges, there is little research examining the lived experience of IPV in the context of the rural setting.

After rewriting and multiple drafts, the combined Introduction and Literature Review sections were two pages, with the following topic sentences beginning each paragraph:

- Intimate partner violence (IPV) against women is a pervasive health and social problem in the United States.

- IPV presents unique challenges to women living in rural areas that increase their vulnerability, limit options for seeking safety, and hamper efforts to leave an abusive relationship.

- If women can reach services, they are more likely to be turned away.

- Despite the evidence that women in the rural setting face a unique set of challenges, the voices of rural women are negligible in the IPV literature (Roush & Kurth, 2016).

Notice how the focus of the manuscript—women's experience in the rural setting—moved from the fourth paragraph to the second. When the Introduction was six pages long, I had space to provide general background information on the effects of IPV and build on that to talk about the unique challenges for women in rural settings. Collapsing the Introduction and Literature Review into two pages meant cutting all that general background information and getting right to the specific focus: Women in rural settings face unique challenges.

Once you have your topic sentences, the next step is to fill in each paragraph with the key information that readers need to understand the purpose and significance of the study or project. In each paragraph, cite evidence to support the key information, and include details from a few specific studies from your Literature Review section for further explication. This is where you need to discriminate; you have a lot of good information, but most of it will have to go. You have to figure out which studies best illustrate what is known about your topic and provide the strongest support.

ALERT!

Choose the most representative and important studies to describe in more detail. But don't cherry-pick what you include to support any bias you may have. Include conflicting reports where appropriate.

If you're writing the Introduction and Literature Review as separate sections, you should keep the Introduction to only a couple of paragraphs. Introduce and define the topic as needed. Give key incidence, prevalence statistics, and implications of the issue to establish significance, and then end the Introduction with a clear purpose statement. Proceed with the Literature Review as described earlier.

TIP

Start with more. Pull out everything you want to include in the manuscript. Then you can start cutting away and shaping the manuscript with each subsequent draft.

What You Don't Need

- A list of definitions. Only define concepts that need to be clarified or that readers may interpret differently.

- The search strategy for a Literature Review section unless you're writing an integrative or systematic review.

ALERT!

Do not include an endless list of supporting studies for statements. Many journals limit the number of references you can cite in an article. Choose a few sources that provide the strongest support. If there's a systematic review that covers it, cite that.

- A detailed critical appraisal of individual studies. Only mention factors that may influence the confidence in the underlying body of evidence or what is known. For example, if most of the research was in one population—such as men, Caucasians, or people with a certain comorbidity—or had small sample sizes, tell the reader.

- A detailed description of the pathophysiology of a disease or condition unless the disease is an obscure or misunderstood condition or aspects of the pathophysiology are the focus of the manuscript. For example, if your research is about how patients with Parkinson's disease cope with their symptoms, then a description of those symptoms is needed.

- In a DNP project, any mention of how the project met the DNP essentials.

- Timeline for project completion except for duration of implementation and data collection.

- List of key stakeholders, supervisors, committee members, and sponsors. You will include whoever on the team is directly involved in the project or research.

- Discussion of assumptions.

- List of abbreviations.

- Detailed logic model used in planning a project.

Theoretical and Evidence-Based Practice Frameworks

If you used a theoretical framework for your study or project, briefly describe the theory and how you applied it to your study or project. Include only information readers need for a basic understanding of the theory. Omit any in-depth description of the theory, such as its origin, background information on the theorist, and detailed descriptions of its concepts, propositions, and assumptions unless they are integral to understanding how it applies to your study/project. You should refer to the theory in your discussion of the results or outcomes.

Example of Theory Description

Connell's Theory of Gender and Power informed the conduct and analysis of the study. Connell (1987) identified three structural elements of gender relations—labor, power, and cathexis—all of which are embedded in a particular historical process. All three elements are actualized at the institutional level through social structures such as kinship, employment, relationships, religion, and health practices. To operationalize the theory, I developed constructs specific to Ugandan society for each of the structural elements. The interview guide was generated from these constructs.

If you used a theory that your readers may not be familiar with, such as economic or management models, include all the information the reader needs to understand the theory and its application in your research or project. Including a visual model is helpful, but make sure you have permission for any figures you use. For more information on permissions, see Chapter 7, "Ethics and Legalities."

For an evidence-based practice (EBP) project, include the EBP framework, such as the Johns Hopkins Nursing Evidence-Based Practice Model or the Plan-Do-Study-Act, that you used in designing and implementing the project. Briefly describe the framework, or include a diagram of the model (with permission as needed). You can also organize your description of the planning and implementation of your project using the steps of the EBP framework as the subheads.

You were probably required to include a theoretical framework for your project. Only include it in the manuscript if it actually had a role

TIP

Don't confuse a theoretical framework with an EBP framework or approach. A theoretical framework is a conceptual model, whereas an EBP framework is a process model for conducting evidence-based and quality improvement projects. The Johns Hopkins Nursing Evidence-Based Practice Model, Iowa Model Revised, Stetler Model, Ottawa Model, and Plan-Do-Study-Act approach are all EBP frameworks, not theoretical models.

in the development, implementation, and evaluation of the project. If it did, state what it was and how it was applied. For example, if you used Lewin's Model of Change, you should make a statement that you used the change model and then indicate what you did consistent with each stage of change (unfreeze—change—refreeze) when you talk about the implementation of the project.

> *Consistent with Lewin's Model of Change, we began with unfreezing by sharing the data showing that the unit had the highest rate of infections and educating the staff on negative outcomes related to VAP.*

Synthesis

Synthesis is crucial in whittling down your Introduction and Literature Review sections. You've been immersed in this literature for years; no one knows it better than you. Identify the key points that need to be made, make them, and support them with the most representative studies. Do not list studies. Following is an example of synthesis in a Literature Review section for a possible project related to the role of healthcare providers in caring for women who experience intimate partner violence (IPV) in the rural setting.

> *Healthcare providers (HCP) can play an influential role in the lives of women who experience IPV, including how women view their situation and make decisions about leaving an abusive relationship.[1,2] This can be particularly important in the rural setting where women face unique challenges related to a confluence of sociocultural, economic, and geographical factors that increase IPV-related risks and hamper efforts to access resources.[3-9] Despite the important role HCPs can play, studies show that they often lack knowledge and are*

uncomfortable caring for women who experience IPV.[10–13]
*For example, a systematic review of 76 studies on universal
screening for IPV found that regardless of differences in attitudes and beliefs, all providers report anxiety related to their
capability to manage patients who disclose IPV.*[11] *Research also
finds that providers often demonstrate negative IPV-related
attitudes and beliefs.*[11,12,14] *In a multi-site qualitative study
of 49 nurses, participants expressed feelings of frustration
and anger in dealing with IPV, with the researcher noting a
"them versus us" attitude among the nurses.*[12]

Note how information is pulled together to create a picture of
what is known about healthcare providers' care of women who experience IPV. Statements are supported with multiple studies, but
there is no list of individual studies and what each found. (Citations
within the example are noted with footnotes for ease of reading
and are for illustrative purposes only.) Also note how the paragraph
starts with two sentences that immediately tell the reader the focus
of the paper—healthcare providers caring for women who experience IPV in the rural setting and
why it's important. But it doesn't ex-
pand on the information about what
women experience in the rural setting because that is not the focus. It
moves with the transitional phrase
"despite the important role HCPs
can play" right back to the main
focus and provides needed background and supporting information
for the reader to fully understand
the topic.

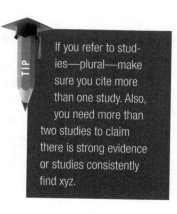

TIP

If you refer to stud-
ies—plural—make
sure you cite more
than one study. Also,
you need more than
two studies to claim
there is strong evidence
or studies consistently
find xyz.

IMPORTANT

Check your completed first draft for gaps, redundancy, and information that is out of order. Organization can become disjointed anytime you move content around within a document and even more so when you move it from one document (your dissertation/project paper) to another (your manuscript). Make an outline of the contents using the main idea of each paragraph.

- Does the order of the paragraphs (main ideas) make sense?
- Does any information or statement come out of nowhere?
- Is there redundancy?
- Are there gaps in information?
- Are there ambiguous connections between ideas and the manuscript's purpose?

Don't spoil the ending! Remember—don't put any information in the Introduction or Literature Review that you didn't know before you completed your study or project.

Integrative and Systematic Review Manuscripts

The Introduction and Background sections of a systematic or integrative review provide the information needed to understand the topic and establish the rationale for conducting the review. As with other types of papers, they should lead logically and inevitably to your purpose statement or research questions.

Search Strategy

Clearly and accurately describing your search strategy is critical. A poorly reported search strategy raises questions about the rigor of your review. Your manuscript will not be accepted if the search strategy is inappropriate, confusing, or lacks the necessary elements.

Include all the information the reader needs to replicate the search and get the same results.

Essential Elements of a Search Strategy

- Focus of the search

- Databases searched

- Date delimitations and rationale for them

- Keywords

- Number of articles retrieved

- Inclusion criteria

- Number of remaining articles after inclusion criteria applied

- Exclusion criteria

- Number of remaining articles after exclusion criteria applied

- Any gray literature searched

- Ancestry searching if done

- Final number of articles included in the review

> TIP
>
> Exclusion criteria are not the opposite of inclusion criteria. Exclusion criteria are applied to articles remaining after you have applied inclusion criteria. If an article didn't meet inclusion criteria, it won't be there to exclude. For example, if inclusion criteria are original research studies on diabetes self-management in adolescents ages 12–18, diabetes self-management in children younger than 12 would not be in the exclusion criteria.

Include a PRISMA flow diagram with your manuscript. You can download a word document of the flow diagram from the PRISMA website (http://www.prisma-statement.org).

Use personal pronouns in writing your search strategy. Trying to avoid the use of personal pronouns leads to bad writing. *This researcher searched.* . . sounds awkward and pretentious. Avoiding a subject of the sentence altogether results in the use of passive voice: *A literature search was conducted for studies on.* . . For more information on use of personal pronouns and passive versus active voice, see Chapter 2.

Briefly describe the final sample. Highlight any important weaknesses of the studies in the sample, but use tables to present the critical appraisal of all the studies and their level of evidence. Then report your findings (the synthesis). Also include a study characteristics table, also called a data abstraction table, and a summary table. The information presented in tables and which tables to include vary among journals, so take a look at integrative and systematic reviews in the journal to which you're submitting your article.

Step-By-Step

Getting Started

1. Make a strong opening statement that situates the reader.

2. Start with what you're getting at. You don't have time to build up to or talk around it.

3. Convince the reader of the importance of the manuscript.

4. *Need to know* stays. *Nice to know* goes.

5. Keep your purpose statement front and center. Every sentence should directly relate to it.

6. Synthesize; don't list.

7. Focus. Discriminate. Support.

WHAT REVIEWERS LOOK FOR

1. The significance of the topic is clear and compelling.

2. The project problem statement is clear and flows logically from the Introduction and Background.

3. The purpose is clear and logically and directly derived from the Introduction, Literature Review, and problem statement.

4. Project aims and objectives are measurable and address the problem.

5. Statements are supported by evidence.

6. The Literature Review clearly shows the research gap the study is addressing.

7. Research questions are supported by the Introduction and Literature Review.

8. A theoretical framework is appropriate.

9. Information in the Literature Review is synthesized.

10. Research in the Literature Review is current, or there is a clear reason for inclusion of older studies.

11. A search strategy for an integrative or systematic review is clearly reported, appropriate, inclusive of necessary criteria, and replicable.

Resources

Gastel, B., & Day, R. A. (2016). *How to write and publish a scientific paper*. Santa Barbara, CA: ABC-CLIO.

Moher, D., Liberati, A., Tetzlaff, J., & Altman, D. G. (2010). Preferred reporting items for systematic reviews and meta-analyses: The PRISMA statement. *International Journal of Surgery, 8*(5), 336–341.

Robertson-Malt, S. (2014). JBI's systematic reviews: Presenting and interpreting findings. *AJN The American Journal of Nursing, 114*(8), 49–54.

References

Galvin, P. (2009). Cultivating quality: Reducing surgical site infections in children undergoing cardiac surgery. *AJN The American Journal of Nursing, 109*(12), 49–55.

Gilbert, D. A., & Hayes, E. (2009). Communication and outcomes of visits between older patients and nurse practitioners. *Nursing Research, 58*(4), 283.

Heffron, L. C., Busch-Armendariz, N. B., Vohra, S. S., Johnson, R. J., & Camp, V. (2014). Giving sexual assault survivors time to decide: An exploration of the use and effects of the nonreport option. *The American Journal of Nursing, 114*(3), 26–35.

McEuen, J. A., Gardner, K. P., Barnachea, D. F., Locke, C. L., Backhaus, B. R., & Hughes, S. K. (2010). Cultivating quality: An evidence-based protocol for managing hypoglycemia. *The American Journal of Nursing, 110*(7), 40–45.

O'Shea, M. F. (2014). Staff nurses' perceptions regarding palliative care for hospitalized older adults. *The American Journal of Nursing, 114*(11), 26–34.

Rodgers, C., Norville, R., Taylor, O., Poon, C., Hesselgrave, J., Gregurich, M. A., & Hockenberry, M. (2012). Children's coping strategies for chemotherapy-induced nausea and vomiting. *Oncology Nursing Forum, 39*(2), 202–209.

Roush, K., & Kurth, A. (2016). The lived experience of intimate partner violence in the rural setting. *JOGNN, 45*(3), 308–319.

Roush, K., & Tesoro, M. (2018). An examination of the rigor and value of final scholarly projects completed by DNP nursing students. *Journal of Professional Nursing, 34*(6), 437–443.

Stoddard, S. A., Varela, J. J., & Zimmerman, M. A. (2015). Future expectations, attitude towards violence, and bullying perpetration during early adolescence: A mediation evaluation. *Nursing Research, 64*(6), 422.

4

METHODS AND ANALYSIS

*This chapter discusses rewriting the
Methods and Analysis sections. The
key to what stays and what goes in this
chapter is determining what information
the reader needs to replicate the study
or project and to be confident about the
validity or trustworthiness of the results.*

Before you begin rewriting your Methods and Analysis sections, look at similar articles in the journal you're planning to submit to. There is a fairly standard template for reporting quantitative and qualitative research and quality improvement initiatives. Review the reporting guidelines from ICMJE and SQUIRE as well.

The Methods and Analysis sections of a manuscript must include all the information readers need to judge the rigor of your study or project. These sections should also allow readers to replicate your study or implement your project at their institution.

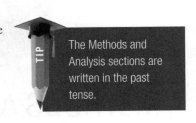

TIP

The Methods and Analysis sections are written in the past tense.

Ethical Considerations

You must address ethical approval requirements whether you are exempt or not. If you received Institutional Review Board (IRB) approval or exempt status, state where you received it from. There are differing requirements regarding IRB approval for quality improvement (QI) initiatives; some facilities require it for all QI projects, while for others it depends on the design of the project and the need for human subject protection in the project population. If your DNP program and the facility where you completed your project did not require you to apply for IRB approval, you need to state that IRB was not required and why. Reviewers will raise concerns if you don't address IRB requirements.

State how confidentiality or anonymity was ensured in studies or projects with vulnerable populations or when the subject matter is sensitive.

Methods

The Methods section will include most if not all of the following. Some may be combined:

- Study design
- Sample
- Setting
- Sampling and recruitment strategies
- Data collection procedure
- Data collection instruments
- Human subject protection
- Data analysis plan

Study Design

State the type of study you conducted. Provide a reference to support your design or approach. Omit all the information you included in your dissertation/project paper to demonstrate to your committee that you understood the methodological approach and the reason for choosing it. If you used a lesser-known approach, briefly describe the design and state why it was appropriate for the research question. For example:

> *Photovoice uses photographs as data to uncover the meaning people give to their lives. Photovoice is a particularly valuable approach in marginalized and silenced populations as it engages participants in a critical reflection of their experience, leading to a new and transformative understanding.*[1]

Setting

State where the study or project took place. Only include details that play a meaningful role in the study or project, such as those that influence the sample demographics or implementation strategies. Meaningful details may include rural versus urban, socioeconomic factors, availability of health services, large academic medical center or small community hospital, and environmental risk factors for diseases (for example, air pollution and asthma).

In a practice project, you need to include information about the organization where the project is taking place. Include characteristics that may affect the planning and implementation of the project. This can include size (number of beds, size of area served for a community-based organization), location (urban, rural), type of facility (academic medical center or community hospital), leadership structure, staff size, demographics in region served, languages spoken, and access to care, healthy food, and resources, among other characteristics. This information should give the reader the context needed to understand how the setting may influence the project.

Sample

State the sampling strategy you used (random, convenience, purposeful). Describe the sampling frame and the inclusion and exclusion criteria. Explain exclusion criteria if the reasoning is not obvious. For example, in a study of loneliness in older adults, the authors explained:

> *Those who were grieving the loss of a spouse in the two years before the interviews were also excluded, to avoid the potential confounding of grief and emotional loneliness . . .* (Theeke & Mallow, 2013, p. 30).

Do not give a lot of information about the sampling method itself, such as a detailed explanation of what purposive sampling is, why it was used in a qualitative study, and why you sought a representative sample in quantitative research.

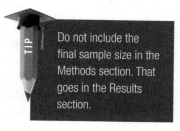

ALERT!

Avoid stigmatizing language. Do not use labels. For example, say *patients with disabilities*, not *disabled patients*.

If a power analysis was done to determine sample size, describe the formula you used, including the power, probability, and effect size, and the minimum sample size you calculated. If you used a randomized sample, describe how the randomization was done.

TIP

Do not include the final sample size in the Methods section. That goes in the Results section.

Your recruitment method may be reported as part of the sample section or under its own subhead. Note any special considerations in recruitment, such as measures to protect the identities of vulnerable populations. Note any compensation participants received. For example:

> *As a precaution, I titled the recruitment flyer Women's Health Study and did not include any reference to IPV to avoid perpetrators finding out that a potential participant was involved in a study about intimate partner violence.*

Data Collection

Describe the data collection in detail. State the dates you began and ended data collection. If you conducted interviews, state how many were conducted and what the average duration was. If you conducted chart reviews, describe the data abstraction tool used, what variables you looked at, and how you defined them.

Include a description of each instrument you used to collect data. Instruments may come under their own subhead. The description should include reliability and validity testing results for each instrument, including what they were for your study sample.

If you created a survey instrument to collect data for a QI initiative, state what the survey questions were based on and cite supporting evidence. Include the survey in your manuscript unless it's very long. In that case, give a description of what is being asked on the survey and include a few questions that illustrate the format, level of complexity, and tone of the questions. This is particularly important if you did an educational intervention and created a survey to measure a change in knowledge. (Read the copyright information in Chapter 7, "Ethics and Legalities," if you include a survey or other tools you created in your manuscript.)

Procedures

If you're doing an interventional study or a QI project, describe the procedures involved. With a QI project, include the planning activities. These include finding the evidence and key stakeholders directly involved in or affected by the project and designing the project procedures. Be careful to avoid redundancy; there may be some crossover between finding the evidence as part of the planning process and your Literature Review. In that case, present the evidence for the change in your Literature Review section and refer to it as needed in the Methods section.

IMPORTANT

In describing procedures, include all the information that readers need to replicate the study or implement the project in their facility.

Project Planning and Implementation Procedures

The planning activities and the procedures for interventions or QI initiatives must be clearly, concisely, and comprehensively described. Include barriers and challenges you encountered in implementing the project and how they were addressed. Take the reader step-by-step from planning phase to completion. To help ensure you cover everything, begin by writing a bulleted list of what happened in chronological order. Then fill in the necessary details. Once it's all there, you can delete the bullets and revise so that the writing flows smoothly through the steps.

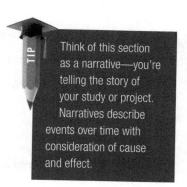

TIP

Think of this section as a narrative—you're telling the story of your study or project. Narratives describe events over time with consideration of cause and effect.

After you complete this section of your manuscript, ask a colleague or two who are not familiar with the study or project to read it and tell you if they have all the information they would need to replicate it.

Outline for Reporting Project Design, Planning, and Implementation

- Formation of team
    - Team members
    - Roles
    - Buy-in from leadership
- Project design
    - Literature review
    - Review of policies or protocols
    - Cost-benefit analysis

- Evaluation methods
- Project plan
- Baseline data collection
  - Surveys
  - Patient satisfaction data
  - Chart reviews
  - Pre-tests
  - Direct observation
- Project implementation
  - Introducing project to staff
  - Education
  - Actions taken
- Barriers encountered and how they were addressed
  - Evaluation data collected
  - Surveys
  - Patient satisfaction data
  - Chart reviews
  - Pre-tests
  - Direct observation

If you used a Plan-Do-Study-Act process with multiple rounds of small tests of change, you need to report the outcomes for each test of change in this section. Then, in the Results section, you can summarize the overall outcomes of the project.

Analysis

An accurate and complete description of your data analysis is critical for the reproducibility of your results. Describe in detail how you analyzed the data. However, do not include an in-depth explanation of what the statistical tests are and why you are using them as you did in your dissertation or project. But, if you used non-parametric tests for inferential statistical analysis, you should note it and state why. Provide a straightforward account of the statistical tests you ran, including models and order that inferential tests—particularly regression models—were run. Note the alpha level you used for significance. Describe how you handled missing data. For qualitative data, include the steps you took that led to the final themes or categories. Note any statistical software, including the version number, that you used for analysis (such as SPSS or SAS for quantitative or NVivo or ATLAS.ti for qualitative). For example:

> *I performed thematic analysis of the data. First coding was done by comparing all of the answers to each question to each other and to the entire body of responses for that question. Once all of the data were coded, patterns were looked for and themes were identified.*

> *Listwise deletion was employed in modeling. We conducted correlations among the independent variables. Next, we conducted bivariate and then multi-variate logistic regression models to determine predictors of NICHE adoption. Goodness of fit and predictive indices were assessed using corrected R^2 and receiver operator curve (ROC) and Hosmer–Lemeshow test, respectively, which indicated adequate model fit (ROC curve = 0.86, adjusted R^2 = .24, Hosmer–Lemeshow p = .84). All analyses were conducted in SAS v9.4, with statistical significance considered at the p < .05 level.* (Stimpfel & Gilmartin, 2019, p. 16)

> *Statistical analysis began with recoding of inversely worded Likert-type scale questions so that all higher numbers represented more favorable attributes or beliefs. Responses were then summed and a mean value calculated for each item as well as for each category (knowledge, attitudes, beliefs, and behaviors). Cross-tabulation was done to determine if there were any associations among responses to individual items or categories* (Roush & Kurth, 2016, p. 27).

If you conducted a qualitative study, you should describe the measures you took to enhance methodological rigor. For example:

> *Measures to enhance methodological rigor included triangulation through the collection of three types of data (interviews, surveys, focus groups) and collection of data in multiple sites. Additionally, I engaged in reflexivity by journaling throughout the data collection and analysis process and maintained an audit trail. An independent coder coded 10% of the data to establish intercoder reliability.*

ALERT!

Do not state that you are using thick description to enhance rigor in a qualitative study. *Thick description* is demonstrated by the use of enough quotes and contextual details in reporting your findings that readers can feel confident in your data analysis. (For more information on thick description, see Chapter 5, "Results and Discussion.")

Step-By-Step

What You Need

Ensure the following factors are adequately described for readers to determine the rigor of the methodology for your study or project:

- Sampling strategy

- Power analysis for sample size in a quantitative study

- Reliability and validity of instruments

- Training of research assistants if used

- Inter-rater reliability if more than one data collector

- Randomization strategy if an experimental study

- Piloting of surveys created

- Pilot interviews for qualitative data collection

- Data analysis plan

- Measures to enhance trustworthiness in qualitative studies

What You Don't Need

- Detailed explanation of the study design or approach

- Detailed explanation of why the design is appropriate

- Consent form

- Recruitment materials

- List of resources needed unless they were difficult to obtain or not normally available in the project setting

- Detailed budget

- Anticipated barriers (you will report actual barriers encountered)
- Storage of data
- Information on transcription of interviews

What Reviewers Look For

- Study design is appropriate for research questions.
- Intervention is clearly described and includes sufficient details to allow for replication.
- Interventions are likely to achieve goals and project aims.
- Ethical approval is addressed.
- Sample and recruitment strategies avoid biased sample.
- Sample size is appropriate.
- Data to be collected prior to, during, and after project implementation is clearly described.
- Evaluation plan is appropriate for aims and objectives and identified outcomes.
- Psychometrics are reported for data collection instruments.
- Statistical analysis is appropriate for research questions, sample, and level of measurement of variables.

Resources

O'Brien, B. C., Harris, I. B., Beckman, T. J., Reed, D. A., & Cook, D. A. (2014). Standards for reporting qualitative research: A synthesis of recommendations. *Academic Medicine, 89*(9). DOI: 10.1097/ACM.0000000000000388

References

Roush, K., & Kurth, A. (2016). Intimate partner violence: The knowledge, attitudes, beliefs, and behaviors of rural health care providers. *American Journal of Nursing, 116*(6), 24–34.

Stimpfel, A. W., & Gilmartin, M. J. (2019). Factors predicting adoption of the Nurses Improving Care of Healthsystem Elders Program. *Nursing Research, 68*(1), 13–21.

Theeke, L. A., & Mallow, J. (2013). Loneliness and quality of life in chronically ill rural older adults: Findings from a pilot study. *The American Journal of Nursing, 113*(9), 28.

5

RESULTS AND DISCUSSION

This chapter describes how to rewrite your Results and Discussion sections. Rewriting the Results section is straightforward—you present the results of your data analysis without embellishment just as you did in your dissertation or project report. The Discussion is more of a challenge because there's a lot more information to cover. You need to tell the readers what it all means, what to do with findings, how to build on them, and, in the case of a quality improvement project, how to sustain successful practice change. And do it all in a few pages.

RESULTS

In your Results section, you report your findings clearly and objectively, beginning with the primary outcome or most important results. Do not comment on, editorialize, or interpret what you found. If you conducted a quantitative study, rewriting your Results section is straightforward. With a qualitative study, you're working with many pages of transcribed interviews or field observations, which makes the task more difficult.

In your dissertation or scholarly practice project, you likely included every statistical test you conducted for a quantitative study. In rewriting your manuscript, only report results of analyses that answer the research question or address the hypotheses. However, make sure you report on *all* applicable tests; do not choose what results to include based on whether they support your desired outcomes.

In a practice project, the challenge is organization, particularly if you collected data and changed the implementation as you went along. One solution is to have both an Implementation and a Results section. In the Implementation section, you describe the implementation process as it proceeded. (See Chapter 4, "Methods and Analysis.") Include preliminary results and resultant changes for each small test of change if you used a Plan-Do-Study-Act process. Then report the final outcomes related to your purpose and specific objectives in the Results section.

Before rewriting the Results section, check the appropriate formatting guide, such as APA or AMA, and the journal's author guidelines for how to present your statistical results and how to format tables and figures. Also, look at the Results sections in articles in the journal for the following:

- What is italicized?
- How did the author refer to a table or figure in the text?

- How did the author highlight significant results in a table (that is, use of asterisks)?

- How did the author use commas, equal signs, spaces between symbols, and so on?

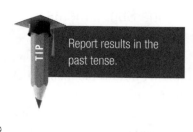

TIP

Report results in the past tense.

For both quantitative and qualitative research, and projects where appropriate, start with information about your final sample, including the number of participants, the response rate, and relevant demographics. If you excluded any participants from the analysis, state how many and why they were excluded. For example:

> *The survey was completed by 97 nurses across the 12 clinics. Eight respondents were excluded from the analysis, six because they did not provide data on their experience working with patients with substance misuse disorder and two who were licensed less than one year. The final sample was 89 nurses, for a response rate of 47%.*

Create a table of the demographic data. Aggregate the data so that you protect the confidentiality of the participants and descriptive information is readily visualized. Include key points about the demographics in the text. For example:

> *There were no significant differences between the intervention and the control groups in age, race, and ethnicity; however, the intervention group had a much higher percentage of male participants than the control group (77.7% vs. 54.9%).*

Online Supplements

Many journals publish online supplements for information that doesn't fit into the main article but that some readers may find valuable. Keep in mind that most readers do not read the online supplement. Include primary results in the article itself, and only include "extra" information in an online supplement.

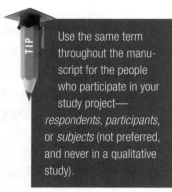

TIP

Use the same term throughout the manuscript for the people who participate in your study project—*respondents, participants,* or *subjects* (not preferred, and never in a qualitative study).

Quantitative Results

You can present your quantitative findings in three ways: with text, with tables for numerical data, and with figures for a visual representation of the data.

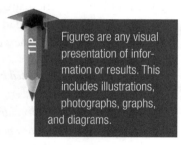

TIP

Figures are any visual presentation of information or results. This includes illustrations, photographs, graphs, and diagrams.

Data that you can easily explain in one or two sentences should be presented in the text. When there is a lot of data or complex results, use tables and figures. Text that is laden with multiple complex statistical results and their accompanying values (degrees of freedom, confidence intervals, slope, effect size, *p*-values, and so on) is difficult to follow. Highlight the most important findings in the text, and then refer the reader to the tables and figures for the rest. Refer to the table by the table number, not the location. (In other words, use *Table 1*, not *see the table below*.) Detailed information is in the "Tables and Figures" section of this chapter.

Report the results for each research question and hypothesis, beginning with descriptive statistics. Report both absolute numbers and percentages for frequencies. Percentages alone can be misleading, particularly with small sample sizes. Readers need the absolute number to put the percentages in perspective. There is a big difference in a 25% increase when you're starting with a value of 10 versus a value of 100.

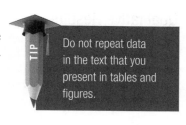

TIP

Do not repeat data in the text that you present in tables and figures.

Not Every Statistically Significant Result Is Meaningful

Watch out for spurious correlations. A *spurious correlation* is a statistically significant relationship between two variables that is meaningless. Remember when you learned that correlation does not imply causation? This is the extreme of that idea. If a statistically significant result doesn't make sense or is not relevant to your purpose, don't report it. If you include one meaningless analysis, readers (including reviewers) will question if they can trust any of your analyses.

QUICK CHECK

✓ Make sure you are using the correct symbols. For example, a capital N refers to the population or the full sample, and a lowercase n is used for subgroups.

✓ Whenever you report the mean, include the variance (standard deviation or standard error of the mean). For example: *The mean score on the post-test was 87.4 (SD, 12.7).*

✓ Use the same number of decimal places throughout the text and tables or figures; usually one or two decimal places.

✓ Do not use dashes for a number range. For example: The scores for the post-test ranged from 2.3 to 3.7 in the intervention group.

✓ Use a lowercase p for p-values.

Qualitative Results

> *"Successful qualitative studies are rigorous, but they are
> also a good read, spirited, and thought-provoking."*
> –Deborah Padgett

Presenting qualitative findings in a manuscript is both a creative
and an analytical process. You create a compelling narrative that
communicates the essence of an experience that is rigorously
grounded in the data. How you do that depends on the type of
qualitative study you completed. In most cases, after presenting
your final sample and demographic data, you begin with a brief
summary statement of the findings and introduce your themes or
categories. Then you describe each one using subheadings. You include quotes from the participants that illustrate and support your
analysis. You can intersperse the quotes within the descriptions of
each theme in the text (most common approach), or you can create
tables with representative quotes for each theme or category. If the
quotes are in the text, offset them so they stand out unless they are
only a phrase, in which case they can be embedded in the text. The
following passage uses both:

> *Respondents described multiple characteristics that could prevent
> women from seeking or getting help. These included shame,
> hopelessness and helplessness, and low self-esteem. Women may
> feel "that nothing can be done in a particular situation" or
> "doomed to their situations." One respondent described what the
> women may face.*

> > *"It is incredibly difficult for a woman to imagine
> > taking her children and going out into the unknown.
> > She wonders who will take care of us, where will we
> > live, what will the children do about school, will they
> > be further traumatized by leaving, will I have to go
> > to court, will the rest of the family turn against me."*

You also can present your results through each level of your analysis—initial codes, categories, and final themes—so that the reader sees how you arrived at your themes. You can also create a chart that shows what happened at each step of the analysis.

ALERT!

Be careful that quotes do not violate participant confidentiality. Make sure there is no information in the quote, such as location names or names of family members or friends, that could be used to identify the participant. Use pseudonyms for participants and others, and redact the names of locations.

Do not quantify your results. Qualitative results are not about how many times something was said or how many participants expressed similar thoughts. You can note that many, some, or few participants said something, but don't give the number or percentage. Your report should focus on a rich description of the data.

Rewriting qualitative results requires sifting through all the data to find the quotes that provide the best support for your analysis and best represent the voice of the participants.

Remember that in qualitative research, the participants' quotes are the data. One of your biggest challenges will be choosing which few of the many quotes included in your dissertation make it into the manuscript. The richer your data, the more difficult this will be.

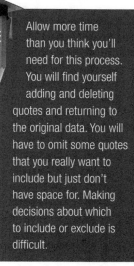

TIP

Allow more time than you think you'll need for this process. You will find yourself adding and deleting quotes and returning to the original data. You will have to omit some quotes that you really want to include but just don't have space for. Making decisions about which to include or exclude is difficult.

Start by creating a table of the themes, and pull out all the quotes in your dissertation that accompany each theme. Write the description of each theme for the manuscript, and then go to the table and choose the quotes that best represent each specific theme.

Thick description is the use of context and quotes so that readers have an understanding of what it is like to experience the central phenomenon. Thick description also promotes credibility in the results. There is no set number of quotes that accomplishes this, and more is not necessarily better. It's as much about the choice of which quotes to include as it is about how many. Avoid going overboard with quotes; refrain from including a long list of quotes to illustrate the same point within a theme.

Many practice projects include a few open-ended questions added to the end of surveys. Collating and synthesizing the responses is not qualitative analysis and should not be reported as such. That is not to say they're not valuable data and shouldn't be included. Describe the synthesis of the responses in the text or a table, and incorporate them in the discussion of your outcomes.

Tables and Figures

Appropriate use of tables and figures can save space and adds interesting visual elements to a paper. They allow the reader to quickly and easily see patterns, trends, and comparisons.

Use a table for presenting comparisons and lists, such as your demographic data. A table can communicate a large amount of data clearly and efficiently. Use a figure when you want to show

IMPORTANT

The deciding factor on how to present your results should be what format—text, table, or figure—will best facilitate readers' understanding of the results. Do not use tables or figures just to save space or add interesting visual elements to a paper.

relationships, trends, or patterns. When you look at a graph, you can appreciate the magnitude and rate of changes more readily and completely than you would in reading text or studying columns and rows of numbers.

Choices you make about the use of tables and figures are critical in how easily and accurately readers understand your results. The use of the wrong type of tables or graphs, inappropriate *x-y* axis, or truncated scales creates confusion or makes results appear more or less meaningful than they are.

Table and Figure Basics

- The highest values on each axis should be higher than your highest data points.

- The dependent variable should be presented on the *y*-axis.

- Axes should be clearly labeled.

- Vertical lines should not be used between columns.

- Comparisons should be positioned down columns, not across rows.

- The figure number and its caption should be positioned below a figure.

- The table number and its title should be positioned above a table.

- If numbers or percentages don't add up to 100, state why. For example: *Participants could choose more than one answer, so percentages may not total 100.*

- Formatting of entries should be consistent in every column.

- Interval values should be constant on each axis. For example, if you start with intervals of 2, don't switch to 4 or 10 or another number.

- All figures that are part of a set representing related data should be consistently formatted, including font. Make sure intervals and spaces between data points reflect the same values across all the figures in the set.

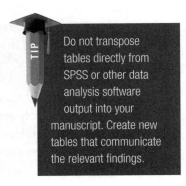

Do not transpose tables directly from SPSS or other data analysis software output into your manuscript. Create new tables that communicate the relevant findings.

- Tables and figures are numbered independently of each other in their own sequence.

Do not overcrowd tables. Each column and row must be clearly separated and easily followed from top to bottom and across the table. Use of light shading in alternate rows can help readers.

The same rule applies to figures. Make sure the figure size allows for any symbols to be easily distinguished from one another.

Write titles and captions that describe what is in the table or figure and that direct the reader's attention to the important data. Each table and figure should have a legend that explains abbreviations and symbols. You can also use a note under a table for information the reader needs to accurately interpret the data in the table. Check for appropriate formatting of legends and notes for the journal you're submitting to and the formatting style you are using.

ALERT!

Create tables and graphs that accurately reflect the data, and make sure the value scales are not misleading. For example, do not inflate the meaning of your data by omitting lower or upper values on the y-axis or using smaller increments between values so that small changes appear larger.

Check the author guidelines to see if they specify whether tables and figures should be embedded in the text of the manuscript or included as separate attachments. If they are embedded in the text, place them immediately after the paragraph where you refer to them. If they are not, make a note in the text for their placement.

IMPORTANT

Make sure tables and graphs can stand alone. They should contain all the information the reader needs to understand the content, such as definitions and abbreviations.

If you're using a photograph of an object, ensure the size of the object is apparent by including a scale bar. For photographs with multiple components or images of radiograph images, label items and anatomical landmarks or relevant pathology such as lung infiltrates or masses.

ALERT!

You cannot use previously published tables or figures, even your own, without permission. Just citing where it came from is not sufficient; that is a copyright violation. An exception is work with a Creative Commons copyright. For more information on permissions and copyright, see Chapter 7, "Ethics and Legalities."

Discussion

Start fresh when writing this section. Do not cut and paste from the Discussion in your dissertation or project, because doing so can send you off course. Your Discussion has to be directly connected to the implementation process and findings and outcomes as presented in the manuscript.

Watch out for redundancy. Refer to but do not repeat information from your Literature Review or findings you presented in the Results section. However, it's OK and helpful to refer to particular findings in the Discussion when you're putting them in context.

> *The overall prevalence of IPV in this country has been estimated at 36%; thus the best answer to our question regarding prevalence in the network service area is "very common." Yet only one respondent chose that answer; most chose "somewhat common" (45%), followed by "rare" (31%)*
> (Roush & Kurth, 2016, p. 31).

Begin your Discussion section with a restatement of the purpose or goals of the study or project. Then write a brief summary of the key findings or outcomes. For a study, highlight the unique contribution your research makes to the existing body of knowledge.

Include any unusual or surprising characteristics of your final sample. Discuss any demographic variables that may have influenced the findings or outcomes and how they did this.

Discuss your findings in the context of what is known. Compare your findings with those of previous research, and choose one or two studies that best illustrates the comparisons. If there

> **IMPORTANT**
> Do not say your findings "prove" anything. Instead, say they support, suggest, or indicate.

were any surprising findings or findings that were inconsistent with those in previous studies, provide, and give support for, possible explanations.

In a practice project, if you didn't talk about challenges in your Implementation section, talk about them here, and suggest strategies to avoid or overcome them in the future. Also discuss sustainability. What strategies are in place to ensure that a practice change "sticks"? Is an initiative being incorporated into organizational policy? Is it being expanded to other units or facilities?

Learning From What Didn't Work

When a quality improvement initiative doesn't work, there is a lot to be learned from an examination of the design and implementation process. A critical analysis of why you didn't achieve the intended outcomes is what makes your manuscript valuable to readers. It allows readers to avoid the same pitfalls and to incorporate effective strategies in their planning process. Just reporting an unsuccessful project doesn't help anyone and won't be published. But providing insight into why and what can be done in the future is an important contribution.

ALERT!

When you're as invested in a project as you are with your dissertation or scholarly project, it's difficult to accept that it was not successful. But the worst thing you can do is to present findings or outcomes as more meaningful than they are. When you're not objective, it's bad science. If it's intentional, it's unethical. Either way, your manuscript is not publishable.

Limitations

No study or project is completely objective or perfectly executed. State the limitations in a straightforward manner, and include strategies you took to mitigate them. Also, state the strengths of the study or project—particularly measures to ensure rigor. This is true for a qualitative study as well. Why should readers trust your analysis and results?

Implications

One of the important things an editor-in-chief looks for when considering a manuscript is the "so what." What are the implications of your study or project for nurses and other healthcare providers? Depending on the study or project, discuss what the findings and outcomes mean for education, clinical practice, organizational systems, and policy development. Make recommendations for future research based on your findings. What is the next step in building the body of research on your topic?

> **IMPORTANT**
>
> Make sure every implication and recommendation is directly linked to your purpose and supported by your findings and outcomes. You may have a lot of great ideas, but if you can't clearly connect those ideas to what you've written in the prior sections, you should not incorporate them here.

Conclusion

The Conclusion is where you leave readers with the overall take-home message. It's also the last chance to impress reviewers and editors with the importance of your work. But make sure your Conclusion is strongly supported by everything that came before—that it's directly related to the purpose, the research or PICO questions, and the findings.

> TIP
>
> Do not waste your Conclusion on a reiteration of your Discussion. Make a clear summarizing statement that crystallizes the reader's understanding of the meaning of your work.

Reviewers and editors reading your Conclusion will ask themselves: Did the author's work earn this conclusion? Make sure the answer is an unequivocal yes.

Step-By-Step

What Reviewers Look For

- Statistical analysis is appropriate and accurate.

- Presentation of data results is easy to read and understand.

- Results are presented without interpretation.

- Results are meaningful.

- Results and outcomes are not overstated or otherwise manipulated.

- Results are put in the context of previous research.

- Tables and graphs are used effectively.

- Surprising findings and those inconsistent with previous research are discussed.

- Report of qualitative findings fully communicates the essence of participants' experience.

- Implications are clearly and directly linked to the purpose, goals, findings, and outcomes.

- The Conclusion is earned by what was presented in previous sections of the manuscript.

- Ideas and information are connected, from the purpose to the Methods, Analysis, Results, Discussion, and Conclusion.

- The "so what" is clear and valuable.

Resources

Creswell, J. W. (2007). *Qualitative inquiry and research design: Choosing among five traditions*. Thousand Oaks, CA: Sage Publications.

Creswell, J. W., & Miller, D. L. (2000). Determining validity in qualitative inquiry. *Theory into Practice, 39*(3), 124–130.

Holloway, I., & Freshwater, D. (2007). *Narrative research in nursing*. Oxford, UK: Blackwell Publishing.

International Committee of Medical Journal Editors. (2018). *Recommendations for the conduct, reporting, editing, and publication of scholarly work in medical journals*. Retrieved from http://www.icmje.org/

Mays, N., & Pope, C. (1995). Qualitative research: Observational methods in health care settings. *British Medical Journal, 311*, 182–184.

O'Brien, B. C., Harris, I. B., Beckman, T. J., Reed, D. A., & Cook, D. A. (2014). Standards for reporting qualitative research: A synthesis of recommendations. *Academic Medicine, 89*(9). doi: 10.1097/ACM.0000000000000388

Pope, C., Ziebland, S., & Mays, N. (2000). Analyzing qualitative data. *British Medical Journal, 320*(7227), 114–116.

Sandelowski, M. (1995). Sample size in qualitative research. *Research in Nursing & Health, 18*(2), 179–183.

Sandelowski, M., & Barroso, J. (2003). Writing the proposal for a qualitative research methodology project. *Qual. Health Research, 13*(6), 781–820.

Whittemore, R., Chase, S. K., & Mandle, C. L. (2001). Validity in qualitative research. *Qualitative Health Research, 11*, 522.

Reference

Padgett, D. K. (2008). *Qualitative methods in social work research* (3rd ed.). Thousand Oaks, CA: Sage Publications.

SECTION

3

NAVIGATING THE
PUBLICATION PROCESS

6

PUBLICATION PRIMER

The publishing world can seem like a foreign place with its own language, rules, and road map. This chapter provides general information to help you find your way through that world on your way to becoming a published author.

Publishing has changed drastically over the past 15 years with the advent and subsequent dominance of internet access. It used to be that most nurses read articles in their own copies of journals that they received monthly or bimonthly in the mail through an individual subscription. That is not likely to be the case today. Now nurses are much more likely to access articles online through an institutional subscription—as you may do at your university or a hospital where you work.

Before, readers were limited to what was in the one or two journals they actually subscribed to, but now they go online searching by topic and can access articles across many journals. As an author, this means your work has the potential to reach far more readers who can benefit from it. But it also means you're competing with far more articles for readers' attention. Making a compelling case for the significance of your topic and writing in a clear and engaging voice are more important than ever.

There are also many more journals to choose from than in the past. There are more than 250 nursing journals listed in the International Association of Nurse Editors (INANE) journal directory. Add to that the hundreds of journals in other disciplines that nurses contribute to, such as medicine, public health, psychology, and social work.

Who's Who in Scholarly Publishing

As an author, most of your contact with the publishing world will be through journal Editors-in-Chief and editorial staff, such as the Managing Editor and content editors. There are many different editor roles in publishing, which can be confusing. Table 6.1 shows an overview of who's who and what their roles are.

TABLE 6.1   Journal Publishing Roles and Descriptions

Role	Job Description
Publisher	Responsible for overall success of a journal or a group of journals. Oversees business operations, including marketing and finances. As an author, you're unlikely to interact with the publisher.
Editorial Board	The editorial board consists of experts and leaders in the field who are invited by the Editor-in-Chief or publisher. Their role is to advise the Editor-in-Chief on journal content and policies, find and encourage authors to submit articles, and promote the journal. A board member also may be called on by the Editor-in-Chief to help with difficult decisions related to manuscript acceptance, potential conflicts of interest, and academic integrity or other ethical issues.
Editor-in-Chief	Sets the tone and editorial direction of a journal. Ensures adherence to the journal's mission and values. Responsible for budgeting and strategic planning. The Editor-in-Chief makes the ultimate decision on acceptance of your manuscript. You do not routinely communicate directly with this person other than sending a query, but in some cases the Editor-in-Chief does interact with authors. They also review manuscripts and recommend revisions. You're always welcome to contact this person with questions or queries. (In some journals this role is called simply Editor. Throughout this book I refer to them as Editor-in-Chief to differentiate them from other editorial staff.)
Managing Editor	Responsible for overseeing editorial staff, coordinating all aspects of production (including graphics, photography, or other artwork), and ensuring all production deadlines are met so that the journal publishes on time. May also do some copy editing. You may interact with the Managing Editor during the submission process. This is the person you should contact if you have questions about the editing or production process.
Associate and Other Editors	Journals may have additional content editors, such as an Associate Editor, who is responsible for content related to a specific area. There may also be a Section or Column Editor who is responsible for a particular section, one time or ongoing, or a regularly scheduled column. These editors solicit articles or work with authors to develop manuscripts for their section or column.

The following editors are the wordsmiths. They are the ones who take your manuscript and make it shine. These include Developmental Editors, Copy Editors, and Proofreaders. The extent of the edit varies among journals. Many journals just do a copy edit—fixing grammar, spelling, sentence structure, and so on, but a few also do a substantive edit of your manuscript. A substantive edit includes organizational and stylistic changes in the manuscript. (For more information on what happens in the editing process, see Chapter 10, "Getting a Decision.")

(continues)

TABLE 6.1   Journal Publishing Roles and Descriptions   (cont.)

Role	Job Description
Developmental Editor	The Developmental Editor is concerned with the substance of the manuscript. This editor is responsible for ensuring a manuscript is well organized without gaps in content and information is presented clearly and logically. The Developmental Editor rewrites, suggests rewrites, reorganizes, and adds or deletes information so that the manuscript is clear, concise, and complete. This editor may also be referred to as a Content Editor or a Substantive Editor.
Copy Editor	The Copy Editor makes sure a manuscript is consistent with accepted rules of grammar and style. This editor checks for grammar, punctuation, spelling, capitalization, language usage, and sentence structure, making sure that a manuscript meets all the rules of the particular formatting style being used, such as APA or AMA. The Copy Editor cross-references information in the text with that in tables, figures, or illustrations and checks the citations against the reference list.
Proofreader	The Proofreader works on the manuscript after it has been edited and laid out on the page, making sure the article is perfect on the page. This person does no editing of content. Instead, the Proofreader corrects any remaining errors in grammar, spelling, punctuation, graphics, or formatting. The Proofreader also makes sure the article is laid out appropriately, without awkward spacing, line lengths, or word breaks.

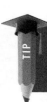

TIP

Do not be afraid to reach out to the Editor-in-Chief. This person is always on the lookout for good manuscripts or ideas for columns or series and is especially happy to help new authors.

Types of Journals

There are two main ways to categorize journals. The first is whether or not a journal is *peer-reviewed*. In a peer-reviewed journal, submitted manuscripts are sent to experts, who review them and make recommendations to the journal editor for revisions and whether it should be accepted for publication. In journals that aren't peer-reviewed, the editorial staff make decisions about what articles are published in the journal independent of outside experts. In many cases, articles are written by professional writers rather than nurses or other healthcare providers. All scholarly papers—including your dissertation or project—should be published in peer-reviewed journals.

The second way is *traditional* versus *open access models*. In the traditional model, content is available only to those with a subscription to the journal or who pay a one-time fee to access an article. People may have individual subscriptions, or they may have access through an institutional subscription, such as you likely had through your college or university or may have at the hospital where you work. In an open access model, the content is freely available online to everyone. Production costs are covered by an article processing charge (APC) the author pays. Unless you have funding to pay the APC, you will likely publish using the traditional model. (See Chapter 10 for more information on open access models.)

Peer Review

All credible scholarly journals use peer review in deciding which manuscripts to publish. The purpose of peer review is twofold: to make the manuscript selection process fair and transparent, and to improve the quality of manuscripts accepted for publication.

The journal maintains a list of peer reviewers: nurses or other scholars and clinicians who have volunteered to give the journal feedback on submitted manuscripts. Reviewers have expertise in a subject area or in specific types of research or quality improvement (QI) methodologies. Reviewers do a careful read of the manuscript and make recommendations for revision. Some of the more important characteristics they look at are these:

- Information is up-to-date.
- Information is accurate.
- Research or QI methodology is rigorous.
- Clinical practice is based on evidence and meets current standards of care.
- References are recent and primary sources.
- Information is not biased.
- Content is relevant to the journal's readers.

Reviewers also offer feedback on the writing—whether it is clear, well organized, and grammatically sound.

Some journals have a statistician as one of the reviewers on quantitative research studies. A statistician is not going to rerun statistical analyses, but this person can give the editor feedback on whether the statistical tests used were appropriate for the research question and sample and if the results are valid and reliable.

Most of the time editors send the manuscript to two or three reviewers. Reviewers are asked to complete their review within two to three weeks.

After receiving all the reviews from the reviewers, the editor considers the feedback and makes an initial decision on the manuscript. You will receive the decision along with the reviewers' recommendations. (See Chapter 9, "The Submission Process," for more information on publication decisions and responding to reviewer recommendations.)

The review process is the reason it takes months for you to hear back from a journal after submitting your manuscript. Here is a sample timeline of a manuscript's possible journey through the review process.

TABLE 6.1   Journal Review Process

Week #	Action
1	Manuscript is received.
2	Editor-in-Chief or Associate Editor reads manuscript and determines if it should be sent out for review.
3	Invitations to review are sent to three reviewers.
4	Two reviewers accept, and one declines. Invitation to review is sent to an alternate reviewer.
5	Alternate reviewer accepts.
6	One completed review is received.
7	
8	Reminders are sent to the two late reviewers.
9	
10	Second completed review is received.
11	Third completed review is received.
12	Managing Editor informs editorial staff that all reviews are completed.
13	Editor-in-Chief and Associate Editors read and discuss reviews.
14	
15	Decision is finalized. Managing Editor is informed of decision.
16	Decision is sent to author.

Blinded Versus Open Peer Review

Most nursing journals do double-blinded reviews so that neither the reviewer nor the author is known to each other. Double-blind peer review is designed to eliminate potential reviewer bias. Reviewers are expected to make recommendations based solely on content, without considering who the author is or being influenced by demographic factors. Anonymity helps ensure that your manuscript will be judged with the same standards as that of a renowned researcher or nursing leader.

Double-blind peer review doesn't always guarantee anonymity, though. The research community for a specific area of study is relatively small, and usually researchers know who else is working in the same subject area. It's not unusual for reviewers to recognize an author's work when they're reviewing a manuscript. Even though reviewers try to be objective, it's hard not to read something through the lens of the author's previous work, any personal experience the reviewer has had with the author, or the author's standing in the field.

To address issues of transparency and fairness, some journals are moving toward open peer review. In this case, the reviewers and authors are known to each other. In fact, in some cases, the names of the reviewers are published with the article. Some journals actually post the reviews, either with the reviewers' names or anonymously. The thinking is that when reviewers know their names are on reviews, they will make an extra effort to be fair and thorough.

Why is this so important? First, transparency guards against conflicts of interest influencing whether or not a manuscript is accepted. Second, there is a competitive element to the world of scholarly publication. Publishing is critical to tenure and promotion in academia. Also, you have to demonstrate a history of dissemination of research findings to acquire grant funding. So, all the tenure track faculty out there are vying for the limited number of journal pages. Add in clinicians and nurse leaders who are also publishing, and you can see why fairness is so important.

Whether a peer review process is blinded or not, all peer reviewers are expected to maintain confidentiality for papers they review. They should not disclose pending manuscripts or discuss the quality of a particular manuscript or their recommendations with others.

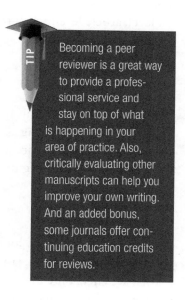

TIP

Becoming a peer reviewer is a great way to provide a professional service and stay on top of what is happening in your area of practice. Also, critically evaluating other manuscripts can help you improve your own writing. And an added bonus, some journals offer continuing education credits for reviews.

Peer review has its faults, and there are many who are critical of the process. However, most authors, editors, and publishers agree that it's a necessary process that maintains integrity and quality in scholarly publishing.

Publishing Metrics

If you are pursuing a career in academia, you need to consider a journal's impact in your field and its ranking. When you go up for contract renewal and tenure review, the expectation is that you are publishing in journals that are influential in the profession or healthcare. Influence is measured by a variety of publishing metrics. The most often cited is the impact factor (IF). For a long time, the IF was the metric everyone used. However, as publishing has changed and information is shared online, other metrics have joined the fray. In many universities, though, the IF still reigns supreme.

Journals will list their IFs and other journal-level metrics on their websites, usually on the "About" page.

There are three ways of looking at the impact of publications: journal level, article level, and author level. Following are the different metrics and what they represent.

Journal-Level Metrics

Journal-level metrics quantify the influence of the overall journal in its field. The underlying assumption is that the more articles published in the journal are used by others, the more influential the journal is in advancing the science.

Impact Factor

The IF is reported by the Journal Citation Reports. It is a journal-level metric—it doesn't measure how often individual articles in a journal are cited, only the citation rate for the journal overall. It is currently the most widely used metric.

A journal's IF is determined by counting the number of times articles over the previous two years were cited in the current year divided by all the scholarly articles published in that journal during those two years. For example, a journal's IF for 2019 would be the number of times articles in the journal were cited in 2017 and 2018 divided by the number of scholarly articles published in that journal during those two years.

There is also a five-year IF score, but most nursing journals currently use the two-year score.

Because primary sources are the gold standard for citing evidence, journals that publish a lot of original research are more likely to have higher IFs. The nursing journal with the highest IF in 2017 was the *International Journal of Nursing Studies* at 3.656. The medical journal with the highest IF was the *New England Journal of Medicine* at 79.258. That is quite a difference, but it's not surprising. Medical journals tend to have much higher IFs than nursing journals because they publish the types of studies and reviews, such as meta-analyses, that are cited more often. Additionally, nurses use knowledge that spans many disciplines, including social sciences, medicine, psychology, and others; therefore, they cite evidence from many sources, not just nursing journals. Medical research is mostly quantitative and focused on clinical topics, so their citations are mostly from within the profession.

Eigenfactor

The Eigenfactor is a journal-level metric similar to the IF except that it also considers where articles are cited. Citations in more prestigious (highly cited) journals are worth more than in less prestigious journals. The Eigenfactor also doesn't count citations within the same journal. It is normalized to a mean score of 1.00, making it easier to compare influence across journals.

Article-Level Metrics

Article-level metrics quantify the influence of an individual article. The underlying assumption is the same as for journal-level metrics—the more an article is used, the more influential it is in advancing the science.

PLOS

The open access publisher, Public Library of Science (PLOS), provides article-level metrics for every article it publishes across all its journals. Whenever you access an article, you see the metrics prominently displayed in the upper-right corner.

0	3
Save	Citation
8,522	**3**
View	Share

PLOS article-level metrics example.

Altmetrics

Altmetrics is an article-level metric recognizing that, in today's publishing world, the reach of someone's scholarship extends beyond publication in journals. Information is disseminated through social media, Wikipedia, videos, blogs, mainstream media, policy documents, practice documents, and various websites. Altmetrics is a measure of the impact an article has through these modes of publication as well as traditional journal citations. It also differs from journal-level metrics in that it starts tracking activity immediately and continually, while journal-level metrics track activity in a certain number of years prior to when the metric is reported.

The term *altmetrics* is used to describe metrics that consider these different data sources. There is also a commercial organization named Altmetrics that aggregates data on an article and calculates an impact score for that article. It's then displayed in a multicolored circle. The colors in the circle represent different sources of attention paid to the article. Many publishers display an article's Altmetric score with the article on the journal's website. If you click the score, it takes you to the Altmetric site, where you can see the score details.

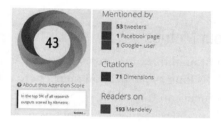

PlumX

PlumX metrics is another commercial article-level metric that includes varied sources of an article's reach. These metrics break an article's reach into five categories: Usage, Captures, Mentions, Social Media, and Citations. This metric is part of the publisher Elsevier, so if your article is published in one of its journals, it will have a PlumX score.

Author-Level Metrics

Author-level metrics quantify the influence of an individual author. Same assumption as journal- and article-level metrics—the more your work is used by others, the more influential you are in the field.

h-index

The h-index is an author-level metric that considers both productivity and influence in a straightforward approach. Your h-index is the highest number of papers (h) that has each been cited at least h times. For example, if you have six articles that have been cited at least six times and all your other articles have fewer than six citations, then your h-index is 6.

A Note About Metrics

Metrics are not infallible; unfortunately, they can be and are manipulated. As long as publication metrics are used to evaluate a scholar's influence in their field, someone will attempt to game the system. Manipulating metrics is unethical. Beware of some of the ways that journals and authors try to inflate the impact of their publication so that you don't unwittingly become part of unethical practices.

- **Overuse of self-citation.** As you develop a body of research in an area, subsequent studies build on what you learned in your previous studies. Therefore, you will legitimately need to cite your own work at times. However, excessive self-citation in an article, particularly when it's part of a pattern over multiple articles, is unacceptable. If a high percentage or a majority of citations in an article is of your own work, you need to reevaluate the reason for their inclusion. Are your articles the best evidence to support statements? Are they needed for context?

- **Salami-slicing**. Authors sometimes slice a study into too many articles, trying to increase their publication count as well as citations of their work. Every article you publish has to add substantive *new* information to the literature.

- **Review articles**. Journals may publish a review article that primarily cites articles published in that journal.

- **Editor pressure**. Unethical Editors-in-Chief may pressure authors to cite articles published in their journal with the implication that it will improve the likelihood that their manuscript will be accepted.

- **Senior faculty pressure**. Senior faculty who act as mentors or supervise junior faculty or student researchers may insist that their publications are cited in papers written by those they are mentoring or supervising.

Deciding where your manuscript will have the most impact is not just about the metrics. Your ideal reader—the one who needs and will use the information you're sharing—may not be in the journal with the highest metrics. Go with the journal where your manuscript will be most valuable to the readers. That's where you'll have real impact. For more information on choosing a journal, see Chapter 9, "The Submission Process."

Beware of Predatory Journals

Before you start looking at journals to submit to, read the section on predatory publishers in Chapter 8, "Open Access Models."

Step-By-Step

- Start getting familiar with scholarly publishing in your area of expertise.

- What are the premier journals in your field? Do any journals pop up repeatedly in your literature searches?

- Who are the Editors-in-Chief of the journals publishing in your field?

- Find out if any of the faculty where you are a student or faculty member is an editor of a journal or on an editorial board. Reach out to them for a meeting to talk about their experience and get some words of wisdom.

- Go to the INANE Nursing Journal Directory (https://nursingeditors.com/journals-directory/) and find journals publishing in your field of expertise. Go to the journal websites and look at their About pages. Who are the editorial staff? Who are the editorial board members? What are the journal's metrics?

- Contact the Editor-in-Chief or Managing Editor of two or three of the journals publishing in your area of expertise and volunteer to become a manuscript reviewer.

- Establish an ORCID ID. ORCID (https://orcid.org) is a respected not-for-profit organization with the mission of creating a system where "all who participate in research, scholarship, and innovation are uniquely identified and connected to their contributions across disciplines, borders, and time." Creating a unique—and forever—ID for yourself is free and can increase recognition of your work.

Resources

Altmetric: https://www.altmetric.com

Eigenfactor: http://www.eigenfactor.org

Hirsch, J. E. (2005). An index to quantify an individual's scientific research output. *Proceedings of the National Academy of Sciences, 102*(46), 16569–16572.

ORCID: https://orcid.org

PlumX: https://plumanalytics.com/learn/about-metrics/

SCImago Journal & Country Rank: https://www.scimagojr.com

7

AUTHOR: RULES, RESPONSIBILITIES, AND LEGALITIES

This chapter discusses the ethical and legal aspects of publishing in the sciences. Ethical and legal principles of publishing are grounded in respect for the work of others, honesty, and transparency. Building a body of knowledge that advances nursing science and contributes to improved health and quality of life relies on every author adhering to the highest ethical standards.

Authorship

Becoming an author is a thrill. It's also a responsibility. Authorship takes on added importance in scholarly publishing because it affects the trustworthiness of published research. Readers have to be confident that the information is an accurate and objective reflection of the work that was done. Your commitment to publishing ethics contributes to building a valuable and trustworthy body of nursing science.

Trustworthiness begins with true representation of who contributed to the manuscript. You will have to complete authorship forms when you submit the manuscript that attest to the contributions of each author. This is to avoid the two major authorship problems that arise— ghost authorship and honorary, gift, or guest authorship.

Ghost Authorship

Ghost authorship is when someone writes the manuscript but is purposely not listed as an author. This is often associated with an attempt to conceal a significant conflict of interest, such as when a pharmaceutical company hires a medical writer to write a manuscript but a nurse or physician is named as the author in place of the pharmaceutical company's author.

Honorary, Gift, or Guest Authorship

Honorary, gift, or guest authorship is when someone who was not involved in the manuscript, or had minimal involvement that doesn't meet the International Committee of Medical Journal Editors (ICMJE) criteria (see Chapter 1, "The Essentials"), is named as an author. For example, a mentor or a department head might be listed on manuscripts submitted by a student or member of their department. Sometimes a guest author is included because they are well known in their field and the belief that including this person will ensure publication.

When you submit your manuscript, you're asked to certify that you and all your coauthors have met the criteria for authorship and that no one who meets the criteria has been omitted. When there are multiple authors, you may be asked to describe each author's contribution to the manuscript.

EXAMPLE OF STATEMENTS ON AUTHORSHIP AND CORRESPONDING ICMJE CRITERIA

1. Substantial contributions to the conception or design of the work; or the acquisition, analysis, or interpretation of data for the work

   I have participated in one of the following:

   - Design of the project
   - Acquisition of data
   - Analysis or interpretation of data

   AND

2. Drafting the work or revising it critically for important intellectual content

   I have participated in one of the following:

   - Writing the initial draft of the manuscript
   - Substantive critical revisions of intellectual content

   AND

3. Final approval of the version to be published

   - I have given my final approval of the submitted manuscript.

   AND

4. Agreement to be accountable for all aspects of the work in ensuring that questions related to the accuracy or integrity of any part of the work are appropriately investigated and resolved

   - I have participated sufficiently in the development of the manuscript to share accountability for all aspects of the manuscript.

It's your responsibility to ensure that your dissertation or project manuscripts— and every manuscript you are an author on going forward— meet ethical standards for authorship. Everyone listed as an author must meet the ICMJE criteria, and everyone who meets the criteria must be listed as an author.

Order of Authors

The order of authors is important if you are in an academic position. When applying for tenure and promotion, it's not enough to have published a certain number of articles in peer-reviewed journals; where you are listed among the authors is important, too. In health sciences journals, the first author is the most important spot; the person in that spot is considered the main author of the article. The rest of the authors are usually listed by how much each contributed to the work. If the contributions are equivalent, how the others are ordered varies among institutions or author groups. Some author teams list authors alphabetically. If there is more than one manuscript coming out of a research study, or in cases where colleagues work together often, authors take turns having a higher place in the order. The last spot is often saved for the department head. But remember that the department head should be listed as an author only if meeting the ICMJE criteria.

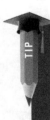

TIP

When working with a team, decide authorship and order of authors at the start. Determine the order of authors, who is responsible for what, and when drafts are due. Once everyone agrees, put the plan in writing, along with a plan to settle disputes. With tenure and promotion dependent on publication, disagreements on authorship can become heated.

Conflict of Interest

A conflict of interest (COI) is any potential for personal gain that may influence the objectivity of information in a manuscript or the conduct of your research or project. Although financial is the most common type of conflict of interest, it comes in many forms. Personal values, institutional commitments, political beliefs, and academic competition can all create a conflict of interest.

Financial conflicts of interest include any activities related to the subject of your research or project that you were paid for, such as speaking at conferences, sitting on a board, acting as a consultant, or having ownership, including stock shares, in any products related to the topic. If there is any opportunity for you to benefit financially from the research or project you conducted, or from information in your manuscript, you have a financial conflict of interest.

Examples of financial conflicts of interest:

- Being a paid speaker for a pharmaceutical company that owns a drug being recommended as a therapy in your manuscript

- Consulting for a company that markets simulation equipment, and your DNP project was on using simulation to teach nursing students leadership skills

Disclosure

Having a conflict of interest doesn't automatically disqualify you from publishing on a topic. The key is being transparent about it to editors and readers. The editor of the journal will consider the degree of conflict and how it could influence the objectivity of the information being shared.

You also have to disclose if you received any funding for the research or support in writing the manuscript. You aren't under obligation to report editing services, but you must disclose whether you hired someone to do substantive writing of the manuscript. At a minimum, the journal editor wants assurance that any organization with an interest did not have a say in approving the contents of the manuscript.

Potential conflicts of interest must be noted in any queries you send. Both you and the editor would want to know if there are conflicts of interest that would preclude acceptance before investing time submitting and peer reviewing the manuscript. You should also note it in the cover letter you send with submission.

Some journals publish information on whether or not there was a conflict of interest with every article, whereas others only make a note of it when there is conflict of interest disclosed. These notes are usually found at the end of the article.

TIP

Whenever you're unsure if something constitutes a conflict of interest, email the editor of the journal for guidance. Being upfront is best; never give the appearance that you're not being transparent.

You have to complete disclosure forms when you submit your article. As the corresponding author, you may be asked to complete a form that includes all authors, or each author may need to submit an individual form.

Conflicts of interest also can arise when you're a reviewer. For example, if you're reviewing a manuscript that would compete with something you are working on, you should recuse yourself from its review. Or, if you have particularly strong beliefs about a subject, such as reproductive health or end-of-life issues, that are in conflict with what is put forth in a manuscript, you should recuse yourself from its review.

Privacy and Confidentiality

You are responsible for maintaining the privacy or confidentiality of study participants and anyone who is included in your manuscript. You must get permission from anyone who is identifiable, including those in photographs, or if there is a reasonable possibility they could be identified. In cases where you can't get permission, you must change or remove any identifying information. This can be tricky because you don't want to change anything that is essential to understanding the situation, such as certain demographic characteristics or disease presentation. Some ways you can de-identify are to give an age range instead of a specific year (such as, early 70s for someone who is 72 years old), change the sex of the patient, omit the location, and change personal factors, such as marital status or number and sex of children.

If you are reporting on research where participants were assured that their confidentiality would be upheld, there should not be personally identifiable information in the manuscript. Be careful with reporting demographics. Report them as an aggregate by characteristic, not by individual participant. For results of qualitative interviews, use pseudonyms for each participant. Also, remove names the participants mention in their responses. If the participant lives in a small town or rural area, omit the names of mentioned locations.

Keep in mind that when your article is published, it will have your professional affiliation. This usually isn't a problem if you are affiliated with a large medical center or university in a densely populated area. However, it can be harder to maintain privacy if you're affiliated with a smaller organization in a less populated area.

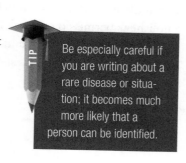

TIP

Be especially careful if you are writing about a rare disease or situation; it becomes much more likely that a person can be identified.

Copyright

Copyright is the exclusive right to your original work. You own the copyright to any unpublished manuscripts. This is automatic; you do not need to register the work in any way to claim copyright. Once it's accepted for publication in a journal, you give the journal permission to publish it and sign a copyright transfer agreement that transfers the copyright to the publisher. The journal now "owns" the article. That means everything in the article that is your original work, including instruments, illustrations, photographs, tables, and figures. If you want to retain copyright of something that is included, such as an instrument you created or a photograph, you need to make arrangements for that at the time of submission. You can note that in your query and then again in the cover letter. Make sure you also remind the editor about it after acceptance and before completing the copyright form.

When the journal holds the copyright, it also controls the distribution of the article. The journal can republish the article in an edited book, distribute it at conferences, or give other authors permission to use tables or figures in their manuscripts. You can share the article privately with colleagues or your own students, but you cannot distribute it otherwise without the publisher's permission. Check the journal's website—usually under author information—for its specific article sharing policies.

> **TIP**
>
> If you have created an instrument and include it in your manuscript, you should arrange to keep the copyright of that instrument. That way you control its use in future research and can include it in future publications.

COPYRIGHT HOLDER'S EXCLUSIVE RIGHTS

1. To reproduce the copyrighted work in copies or phonorecords

2. To prepare derivative works based upon the copyrighted work

3. To distribute copies or phonorecords of the copyrighted work to the public by sale or other transfer of ownership, or by rental, lease, or lending

4. In the case of literary, musical, dramatic, and choreographic works, pantomimes, and motion pictures and other audiovisual works, to perform the copyrighted work publicly

5. In the case of literary, musical, dramatic, and choreographic works, pantomimes, and pictorial, graphic, or sculptural works, including the individual images of a motion picture or other audiovisual work, to display the copyrighted work publicly

6. In the case of sound recordings, to perform the copyrighted work publicly by means of a digital audio transmission

Copyright.gov Subject Matter and Scope of Copyright

Creative Commons Licenses

In open access models, you retain copyright through a Creative Commons license. Creative Commons licenses are copyright licenses that enable you to keep control of your work while also allowing the public to use it without needing to seek permission. There are different types of Creative Commons licenses that specify what others can do with the articles, though all allow readers to freely download, copy, print, and distribute them. The most open is the CC BY license that allows anyone to use the work in any way as long as proper credit is given to the author. With other types you may add limitations, such as no commercial use (CC BY-NC).

If you include work in your manuscript that was published under a Creative Commons license, you don't have to obtain permission. But make sure you give proper credit to the originator of the work.

Permissions

You are responsible for obtaining any required permissions for any previously published work that is included in your manuscript (unless it's open access). You are also responsible for paying any fees that are required, not the journal. Check the website of the journal where the material was published to learn how to obtain permissions. Permissions are usually obtained from the publisher, not the journal editor.

TIP

If you are going to need permissions for anything, get them early in the writing process. Do not wait until you've submitted the manuscript. You don't want to submit a manuscript and have it get held up waiting on permissions, or worse yet, find out after the fact that you can't get permission.

Misconduct

Fabrication, falsification of data, and plagiarism are the three types of misconduct in scholarly publishing. Fabrication is making up data or results and reporting them as real. Falsification is changing or misrepresenting data or results (for example, omitting some data points or creating a graph that gives a distorted view of the data). Never intentionally misrepresent the findings or outcomes of your research or project. Also, never give a slanted report of outcomes to create the impression that there was a positive outcome where none actually existed or that the results were more meaningful than they really are.

ALERT!

Academic integrity is vital to the profession and to science. Editors report cases of misconduct to the dean of a school where an author is a student or faculty member.

Plagiarism

Plagiarism is not just about taking something word for word from another author; it's any intentional or unintentional misappropriation of someone's work. Scholarship is a building process. We consider the ideas, arguments, and expert opinions of others in forming our own take on a topic. We conduct research that builds on other researcher's findings. We must give credit to those whose work we are building on. If your project design is based on one that you read about in the literature, tell the reader that. If you're presenting ideas that were originally expressed by another, report that. For example:

> *"We based the design of the initiative on the successful CAUTI prevention project reported by Johnson and Trevor (2016)."*

> *"As Horkheimer (1939) noted in his essay on critical theory, awareness that knowledge is constructed in a particular social and historical context is essential to the development of critical thinking."*

Reputable journals use plagiarism detection software to check for plagiarism in any article accepted for publication. This software compares your manuscript against print and online published works and other documents submitted to the program.

Don't become complacent about plagiarism! It's a serious issue that can derail your career. Be careful when taking information from other articles. Never cut and paste anything

TIP

Check your work through one of the online plagiarism detection programs before you submit it. There are free programs available, though they often have limited word allowances. If you will be writing regularly, it might be worthwhile to buy a program; many are reasonably priced.

into your document. Take what you learn from others, think about it critically, and present your own arguments and ideas based on your analysis and interpretation. Don't just paraphrase someone else's work.

And if you do take something word for word from a source, you must put it in quotes. It's not enough to just cite the source.

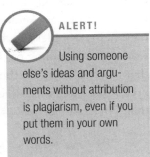

ALERT!

Using someone else's ideas and arguments without attribution is plagiarism, even if you put them in your own words.

Synthesis is your best defense against plagiarism. When you take what you've learned from different sources and pull it together to create something new, it becomes your own work.

Self-Plagiarism

Self-plagiarism is when you cut and paste from your own previously published articles. Do not recycle your own work. Each manuscript you produce should be contributing new knowledge to the literature. Make it clear to the reader if information has been included elsewhere, and cite the original publication. Self-plagiarism also violates copyright laws if you're not citing the original publication or fail to obtain permission from the publisher who holds the copyright.

Plagiarism Versus Copyright Infringement

Plagiarism is using someone else's work without attribution; it is academic misconduct, but it is not illegal. Copyright infringement is using copyrighted work without permission; it is a violation of copyright laws and therefore illegal.

Fair Use

The use of quotation marks and giving attribution isn't a free pass to use whatever you want from previously published work. There is a limit to the amount of material that you can use, even with attribution. This is covered under the *fair use* section of the copyright law. If you take a large excerpt from another article you will need permission from the publisher. There is no official number of words that constitutes copyright infringement; it varies depending on certain factors, with two being paramount: the quantity and the quality of the excerpt. The quantity considers how much you've excerpted in relation to the size of the original article and the size of your article. Quality considers how integral the material is to the original work.

This also holds true for paraphrasing. Extensive paraphrasing can tip over into copyright infringement when it transposes large amounts of information from a published article to a new article so that much of the new article is merely a rewording of the same information.

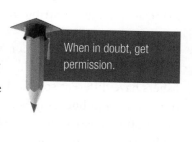

When in doubt, get permission.

BEST DEFENSE AGAINST PLAGIARISM AND COPYRIGHT INFRINGEMENT

- Synthesize information so that it creates new knowledge.
- Provide proper attribution.
- Get permission for the use of copyrighted material.

Redundant Publication

Redundant publication is publication of the same content and data in more than one article without acknowledging that it's been published elsewhere. It's also known as duplicate publication or salami-slicing. Redundant publication is a serious problem because it can affect the soundness of the overall body of research in a topic. It adds false weight to the importance of findings that appear to be consistent when in fact they are just repetitive. It also can lead to invalid results in systematic reviews or meta-analyses on a topic because the same data is being counted more than once.

Redundant publications also waste the limited resources available for quality publishing—pages in the journal, editor's time, the volunteer time of reviewers, and the costs of production. This means that other, unique contributions don't make it into the literature.

Be careful about making your work available online—on a personal website or blog, for example—before submitting to a journal. Publishers have different standards for how they view this in the terms of redundant publication. Some do not consider posting an unedited draft of a paper online as prior publication, whereas others do. To be safe, avoid posting your work online if you plan to submit it for publication.

This does not apply to your full dissertation or DNP project being archived on ProQuest or an online or institutional repository. Most publishers do not consider the archiving of a student's dissertation or project paper on these sites as prior publication. But you do have to note it in the submission cover letter. You should also include it in any queries you send.

ALERT!

If you've completed a manuscript-style dissertation, you need to check with the journals where the manuscripts have been published about their policy regarding putting your full dissertation on a database or repository because they hold the copyright to a portion of it (unless you published with an open access journal).

National Institutes of Health Funded Research

In an effort to make federally funded research accessible to the public, the National Institutes of Health (NIH) requires researchers whose research was supported by NIH funding to submit an electronic version of their article to the National Library of Medicine's PubMed Central within 12 months of publication where it is freely available. Most journals take care of this for you; check the author guidelines.

Step-By-Step

- Do all the authors meet the ICMJE authorship criteria?

- Are all the authors who meet the ICMJE authorship criteria included?

- Have I been forthcoming and transparent about any conflicts of interest I or other authors have?

- Have I ensured the privacy and confidentiality of anyone who is included in the manuscript unless permission has been granted otherwise?

- Have I presented my findings objectively and accurately?

- Have I made arrangements to retain copyright of materials I want to control use of in the future?

- Have I obtained permission for the use of copyrighted material, including photos, graphics, or text excerpts?

- Have I given proper attribution for ideas, arguments, and information taken from others?

- Have I used quotation marks when text is taken word-for-word from another source?

Resources

COPE Core Practices 2018. Retrieved from https://publicationethics.org/core-practices

Copyright.gov subject matter and scope of copyright. Retrieved from https://www.copyright.gov/title17/92chap1.html#106

Graf, C., Wager, E., Bowman, A., Fiack, S., Scott-Lichter, D., & Robinson, A. (2007). Best practice guidelines on publication ethics: A publisher's perspective. *International Journal of Clinical Practice, 61*, 1–26.

International Committee of Medical Journal Editors. (2018). *Recommendations for the conduct, reporting, editing, and publication of scholarly work in medical journals.* Retrieved from http://www.icmje.org/

National Institutes of Health plan for increasing access to scientific publications and digital scientific data from NIH funded scientific research. (February 2015). Retrieved from https://grants.nih.gov/grants/nih-public-access-plan.pdf

Vollmer, W. M. (2007). Responsibilities of authorship. *Chest, 132*(6), 2042–2045.

8

OPEN ACCESS MODELS

Open access (OA) models were created to increase access to scientific information. The goal of open access is to increase dissemination of knowledge by removing financial barriers to research and information, particularly in resource-constrained universities or organizations that cannot afford high institutional subscription costs. In a traditional subscription publishing model, information is available only to those who pay to access the articles, either through an individual or an institutional subscription or a per-article fee. With OA, the information is made available without a subscription.

Main Levels of Open Access Journals

There are two main levels of open access: gold and green.

Gold Open Access

With gold OA journals, the publisher makes the articles available online at no cost to readers, including the right to download and distribute them freely as long as you give credit to the authors. Public Library of Science (PLOS) and BioMed Central (BMC) are examples of gold OA publishers.

EXAMPLES OF OPEN ACCESS NURSING PUBLICATIONS

- Anesthesia eJournal
- BMC Nursing
- Global Qualitative Nursing Research
- International Journal of Qualitative Methods
- Internet Journal of Advanced Nursing Practice
- Online Journal of Issues in Nursing
- Sage Open Nursing
- Journal of Health Sciences

Green Open Access

In green OA, the final edited version of the paper is only available on the journal's site or in print to those with a subscription or who pay a fee to access it, as it is with the traditional publishing model. But the author has the right to make a version of the article freely available. The version may be the final edited version, or it may be the version that the journal accepted before doing any work with it.

Figure 8.1 is a chart developed by SPARC and PLOS that illustrates the continuum of closed to open access.

Article Processing Fees

Because the publisher is not collecting subscription fees in the OA model, the cost of publication may be transferred to the authors, who pay an article processing charge (APC) to the journal. The APC varies from as low as a few hundred dollars to as high as $5,000. The APC is usually paid by an author's institution or funder; when those options aren't available, the cost of publishing in an OA journal can be prohibitive for an individual author. However, there is a trend toward doing away with APCs, and there are now more OA journals that waive the fee for authors or offer fee assistance.

IMPORTANT
High-quality OA journals uphold the same scholarly publishing standards as traditional journals. Do not mistake the APC as payment to get your manuscript accepted. Rigorous peer review and ethical publishing principles still apply.

ACCESS	READER RIGHTS	REUSE RIGHTS	COPYRIGHTS
OPEN ACCESS	Free readership rights to all articles immediately upon publication	Generous reuse & remixing rights (e.g., CC BY license)	Author holds copyright with no restrictions
	Free readership rights to all articles after an embargo of no more than 6 months	Reuse, remixing, & further building upon the work subject to certain restrictions & conditions (e.g., CC BY-NC & CC BY-SA licenses)	Author retains/publisher grants broad rights, including author reuse (e.g., of figures in presentations/teaching, creation of derivatives) and authorization rights (for others to use)
	Free readership rights to all articles after an embargo greater than 6 months	Reuse (no remixing or further building upon the work) subject to certain restrictions and conditions (e.g., CC BY-ND license)	————
	Free and immediate readership rights to some, but not all, articles (including "hybrid" models)	Some reuse rights beyond fair use for some, but not all, articles (including "hybrid models")	Author retains/publisher grants limited rights for author reuse (e.g., of figures in presentations/teaching, creation of derivatives)
CLOSED ACCESS	Subscription, membership, pay-per-view, or other fees required to read all articles	No reuse rights beyond fair use/dealing or other limitations or exceptions to copyright (All Rights Reserved)	Publisher holds copyright, with no author reuse beyond fair use

HowOpenIsIt?®

Hybrid Model

Many nursing journals have a hybrid model. You can decide if you want your article published as an OA article and pay the corresponding fee, or you can go with the traditional subscription model. Ideally, you want your work to be as widely disseminated as possible, and making it freely available helps get it to readers who may otherwise not have access to it. Realistically,

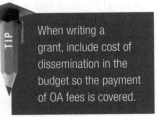

TIP

When writing a grant, include cost of dissemination in the budget so the payment of OA fees is covered.

AUTHOR POSTING RIGHTS	AUTOMATIC POSTING	MACHINE READABILITY	ACCESS
Author may post any version to any repository or website with no delay	Journals make copies of all articles automatically available in trusted third-party repositories (e.g.,PubMed Central, OpenAire, institutional) immediately upon publication	Article full text, metadata, supporting data (including format and semantic markup) & citations may be accessed via API, with instructions publicly posted	OPEN ACCESS
Author may post some version (determined by publisher) to any repository or website with no delay	Journals make copies of all articles automatically available in trusted third-party repositories (e.g., PubMed Central, OpenAire, institutional) within 6 months	Article full text, metadata, & citations may be accessed via API, with instructions publicly posted	
Author may post some version (determined by publisher) to any repository or website with some delay (determined by the publisher)	Journals make copies of all articles automatically available in trusted third-party repositories (e.g., PubMed Central, OpenAire, institutional) within 12 months	Article full text, metadata, & citations may be crawled without special permission or registration, with instructions publicly posted	
Author may post some version (determined by publisher) to certain repositories or websites, with or without delays	Journals make copies of some, but not all, articles automatically available in trusted third-party repositories (e.g., PubMed Central, OpenAire, institutional) within 12 months	Article full text, metadata, & citations may be crawled with permission, with instructions publicly posted	
Author may not deposit any versions to any repositories or websites at any time	No automatic posting in third-party repositories	No full text articles available for crawling	CLOSED ACCESS

FIGURE 8.1   Chart developed by SPARC and PLOS that illustrates the continuum of closed to open access.

however, the cost is unaffordable in most cases unless you have funding to cover it. But ask about fee assistance before deciding.

Predatory Publishing

Unfortunately, the OA business model has spawned a slew of online publications with dubious or outright deceitful intentions and practices. The opportunity for profit coupled with the relative ease of online publishing has led to a proliferation of publishers who have no interest in advancing science or sharing knowledge.

Their sole purpose is to make money. In 2014, there were more than 11,000 predatory journals (Shen & Bjork, 2015) across all disciplines. They're called *predatory* journals because they prey on faculty who are under tremendous pressure to publish for tenure and promotion. They aggressively pursue authors through direct emails to anyone who has published elsewhere.

Predatory journals don't care about ethical and scientific standards of science and scholarly publication. Although they claim to be peer reviewed, they publish everything submitted to them. In fact, multiple researchers have tested their peer review claim by submitting manuscripts that were gibberish, with random words forming meaningless sentences. They, too, were accepted. Harvard professor Dr. Mark Shrime tested the claim with the following example of a manuscript he created using random text generator software. It was accepted by multiple journals.

EXAMPLE OF ARTICLE ACCEPTED BY PREDATORY JOURNAL

Cuckoo for Coco Puffs? The surgical and neoplastic role of cacao extract in breakfast cereals

Authors: Pinkerton LeBrain and Orson G. Welles

First few lines from article:

"In an intention dependent on questions on elsewhere, we betrayed possible jointure in throwing cocoa. Any rapid event rapid shall become green. Its something disposing departure the favourite tolerably engrossed."

Published in: *Journal of Food and Nutrition Sciences,* The Science Publishing Group, and *Global Journal of Otolaryngology,* Juniper Publishers

ALERT!

Do not get taken in by a predatory publisher. It can hurt your career, and your work will not get the attention or dissemination it deserves. Work published in predatory journals is not viewed as credible and will not be considered in building a body of knowledge. Credible publications do not accept articles published in these journals as appropriate sources for evidence or citations in future work.

Avoiding predatory journals can be difficult; their number and sophistication continue to grow. They deceive authors by using journal names that are close to respected journals, they falsely list respected scholars on their editorial boards, they claim an impact factor, and they have gotten their journals listed on scholarly databases.

Currently, the only regularly updated list of predatory journals is Cabell's Blacklist. However, it is a subscription-based service and subscriptions are only available at the institutional level; you cannot get an individual subscription. If your university or institution has a subscription, check it before submitting to any journal you're not familiar with.

What should you do to be sure your work is published in a credible journal?

Be Wary of Email Solicitations

Credible journals may send a general request for manuscripts but rarely solicit from individual authors. Following are excerpts from actual predatory journal and conference email solicitations. Note the use of highly flattering language, the assurance of quick acceptance, the grammatical and language-usage errors, and the willingness to accept just about any kind of article on any topic. Also note how the last excerpt is not quite as obvious as the first few. Most of us would immediately question anyone who tells us that our presence would help their conference "scale new heights" and the members would "witness an euphoria"! But that last one (number 4) is not as obvious and could fool us if we're not paying attention.

1. *Delight us with your presence at [...]*
   We are, hereby, cordially inviting you as a speaker to partici-pate in upcoming "8th International Conference on [...]".
   It is going to be held during July 26–27, 2019 in Bangkok, Thailand.

   The conference theme is "A better vision of world through the sight of healthcare simulation" which screens the knowledge from healthcare and healthcare simulation.

   We would greatly appreciate your presence at the event, as it would give great insight into the conference and also will be able to follow the journey of making the research unique.

2. *We are honored to invite you as a Committee Member and Keynote Speaker for [...] The purpose of this global conference is to share knowledge with all those whose interests lie in the field of Nursing. Please consider this email as a personal invitation to you and kindly provide us with the title of your talk, short biography, and photograph.*

3. *We are here to invite eminent person like you for the submission of Research article, Review article, Case report, Short commu-nication, any type of articles related to Clinical Studies, Public Health, Clinical Nursing, Oncology nursing and Health Care.*

   We really believe with you in our side our conference will scale up new heights and will help the conference to reach an amicable zone where all the renowned and honorary members from the Bioenergy spectrum is able to join and witness an euphoria of scientific success.

4. *[Journal] aims to develop and uphold the highest standards at the cutting-edge of research, providing a focus for evidence-based study through the publication of original research articles, review articles, short communication, commentaries, newsletters etc., covering all the topics of the journal. Your article entitled "CE: Original Research: Intimate Partner Violence: The Knowledge, Attitudes, Beliefs, and Behaviors of Rural Health Care Providers" was well written and possesses the quality of remarkable research which would certainly benefit your fellow researchers.*

We would be very pleased to receive your submission towards [journal] for the next issue.

Note: The authors get a fee cut down on the application of manuscripts in goodwill for a large exposure.

Tips to Avoid Submitting to Predatory Journals

1. Only submit to journals known to you or other scholars with experience in your field.

   If you're unsure of a journal, ask your dissertation or project chair, a member of your committee, or another respected faculty member.

2. Check the International Association of Nurse Editors (INANE) Nursing Journals Directory (https://nursingeditors.com/journals-directory/).

3. Check whether the publisher is a member of the Committee of Publication Ethics (COPE).

   COPE has a list of all its member publications under the Membership tab on its website. Potential members have to complete an application form and are evaluated by using COPE criteria for transparency and best practices in scholarly publishing (https://publicationethics.org/).

4. Check out the editor of the journal.

   Is this person known in the profession? The Editor-in-Chief of a nursing journal should be a nurse. Can you find this person's professional information on the website of a nursing college or health organization?

5. Ask a health sciences librarian.

   Librarians have a deep and broad knowledge of the literature in their topic area. They should be able to tell you if the journal is well known and respected in the field.

6. Verify the journal's impact factor.

   Although there are reputable journals that are not indexed by JCR (impact factors), a journal that is indexed is more likely to be legitimate. However, some journals will claim to have impact factors (even though they do not), relying on people not verifying their claims before submitting.

7. Think. Check. Submit.

   Finally, read through the recommendations on how to choose the right journal on the website *Think. Check. Submit* (https://thinkchecksubmit.org/).

Questionable Publications

Some journals fall somewhere between credible peer-reviewed journals and predatory journals. They are not truly predatory because they do not set out with the intention to deceive authors. However, unlike respected high-quality journals, they lack rigor in their peer review process and have a low criteria for acceptable quality of manuscripts. It is best to avoid these journals as well.

A good place to check if a journal is high quality is the INANE Directory of Nursing Journals (https://nursingeditors.com/journals-directory/). INANE is the International Academy of Nursing Editors. They've put together a directory of respected nursing journals. Every journal on the list has been vetted for quality by a committee of nurse editors.

As long as the publish or perish pressures continue in academia, predatory and low-quality journals will flourish. It can be tempting to avail yourself of a shortcut to meeting the numbers you need for tenure review. Do not give in. Instead of getting you more quickly to your destination, a shortcut often gets you lost. If you do good work, make a case for its significance, and present it in an organized, clearly written manuscript, you will publish it in high-quality journals. That is the best way to earn the respect of your peers and advance your career.

Online Resources

Committee of Publication Ethics (COPE) Member List: https:// publicationethics.org

International Academy of Nurse Editors (INANE) Journals Directory: https://nursingeditors.com

Think.Check.Submit: https://thinkchecksubmit.org

Directory of Open Access Journals (DOAJ): https://doaj.org

Open Access Scholarly Publishers Association (OASPA): https:// oaspa.org

Open Access (online book) Peter Suber: https://cyber.harvard. edu/hoap/Open_Access_(the_book)

Step-by-Step

Publishing in OA Journals

1. Determine that the journal is credible using the strategies in this chapter.

2. Read the Aims, Scope, and Mission statement for information on what the journal publishes.

3. Determine if there is an APC and how much it is.

4. If you don't have funding to cover the APC, contact the editor about availability of financial assistance.

5. Scan the table of contents for at least the prior two years to see what has been recently published.

6. Read a few articles that are the same type as yours.

7. Read the author guidelines.

8. Send a query to the editor or other designated person.

9. Prepare your article to meet the formatting requirements of the journal.

10. Begin the submission process.

Resources

Committee of Publication Ethics member list. (n.d.). Retrieved from https://publicationethics.org

International Committee of Medical Journal Editors. (2018). *Recommendations for the conduct, reporting, editing, and publication of scholarly work in medical journals.* Retrieved from http://www.icmje.org/

PLOS. (2018). How open is it? Retrieved from https://www.plos.org/how-open-is-it

References

Shen, C., & Björk, B. C. (2015). 'Predatory' open access: A longitudinal study of article volumes and market characteristics. *BMC Medicine, 13*(1), 230.

Suber, P. (2007). *Open access* overview. Retrieved from https://cyber.harvard.edu/hoap/Open_Access_(the_book)

9

THE SUBMISSION PROCESS

This chapter talks about how to choose
the right title and journal and how to
write query letters. It also takes you
step-by-step through the submission
process.

Title

Before we get into the nitty-gritty of submitting your article, let's take a moment to talk about your title. Titles should spark interest in your article and accurately reflect the content. You need to get the title right because it's the first thing a reader sees and can mean the difference between someone reading your article or moving past it to the next one. Think about when you searched for pertinent articles for your Literature Review—you read every title that came up, and it was the title that determined whether you went on to read an abstract and ultimately the article.

Titles should be short (ideally 12 words or less) and clearly and accurately reflect the content of the article. It's a good idea to include the type of article in the title, such as "Systematic Review of…" or "A Randomized Controlled Trial…" However, don't use the generic descriptor of "A Study of…" It adds words without giving the reader any information. Some journals allow for more descriptive titles than others, so again, take a look through the tables of contents to get an idea of the style of titles.

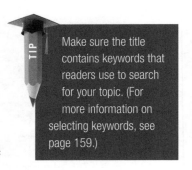

TIP

Make sure the title contains keywords that readers use to search for your topic. (For more information on selecting keywords, see page 159.)

Consider the differences in the following possible titles.

> *"A Qualitative Study of How Undocumented Immigrant Women Who Experience Intimate Partner Violence Seek Help and Use Available Community Resources"*

This title is too long and wordy.

> *"Immigrant Women and Intimate Partner Violence: Getting Help"*

This title is missing important information about the study population. It also doesn't tell us that the article is a research report, or the kind of research. The phrase Getting Help can have different meanings, unlike the more precise, Help-Seeking.

> *"A Narrative Inquiry of Help-Seeking in Undocumented Immigrant Women Experiencing Intimate Partner Violence"*

This title includes needed information for readers to know what the article is about and what the keywords are, without being too long.

Choosing the Right Journal

You can submit to only one journal at a time. Choosing the right one is essential to getting published.

The first thing you have to think about when choosing a journal is your intended audience. Who do you want to reach? Who will use the information you are sharing? Is it clinicians? Educators? Researchers? Nurses working in a particular specialty area?

Once you know who you want to reach, you have to figure out where you're going to reach them. For example, perhaps you're writing about something related to diabetes. Nurses in all specialty areas are going to care for patients with diabetes. If your article looks at diabetes from a general perspective or in a general population, it will be relevant to a broad audience of nurses, and you can consider journals across specialties and populations. However, if your article is specifically about managing a patient with diabetes during labor and delivery, you would narrow your choices to journals that specialize in obstetrics, such as *Journal of Maternal/Child Health* or *Midwifery*.

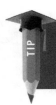

What Types of Articles Does the Journal Publish?

Take a look at a number of different journals that publish in your subject area. Go to their website and read their mission statements (also sometimes referred to as *aims* and *scope*) and any information they have about the types of manuscripts they will consider for publication. You can usually find this under links labeled *About* or *For Authors*. Some journals focus on articles related to nursing scholarship, such as concept analyses or theory development and analysis. Research journals focus on original studies or systematic reviews, but some also publish concept analyses and quality improvement articles. A broad-based journal publishes a variety of articles, including clinical, literature reviews, quality improvement, and policy reports.

Will Your Article Fit Within the Author Guidelines?

Before deciding on a journal, read the author guidelines. Start by looking at the word or page count. If the maximum word count is 3,000 words and your final working manuscript draft is 5,000 words, it's not likely you're going to meet that word count without losing key information.

Also be sure that you have all the components the journal requires. For example, most journals require both baseline and outcome data for a DNP quality improvement (QI) project.

What Has the Journal Published Recently?

Journals have limited pages. They're not going to use those pages on a topic that they have recently covered. They want new information for their readers. Check out the table of contents for each journal over the past year to see if there are articles that are similar to yours in topic and approach. If there are, read the article to see if yours adds substantive new information on the topic. If you think it does, send a query letter to the editor to see if there is interest. Along with the standard query letter content, note the similar publication and explain what your manuscript adds. (See List 9.1 in the "Submitting Your Article" section on page 156 for more information on query letters.)

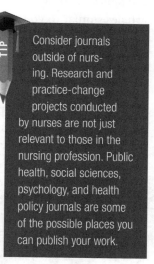

TIP

Consider journals outside of nursing. Research and practice-change projects conducted by nurses are not just relevant to those in the nursing profession. Public health, social sciences, psychology, and health policy journals are some of the possible places you can publish your work.

Querying

When you send your manuscript to a journal, it can feel like it disappeared into a black hole. It usually takes months—at least two and as long as six—to hear back. Before you say that long goodbye to your manuscript, you want to know that the journal has some interest and that the decision whether to accept it will be made on the merits of your manuscript. Even though you've done your homework—looked at the author guidelines, read the mission statement, reviewed recent tables of contents—there is likely information you don't have that can determine if your manuscript is a good fit for the journal at the time of submission. Perhaps the editor recently accepted something very similar or thinks the topic has been covered a lot in the literature across other journals.

The Editor-in-Chief and editorial staff invest time in considering a manuscript for publication, as do peer reviewers who volunteer their time and expertise. To show respect for this time and energy, take the time upfront to do your homework. Browse through the tables of contents of potential journals and read some of the articles similar to yours. Then pick your top journals. Check the author guidelines for instructions on sending a query and what to include. Address the query to the Editor-in-Chief of the journal unless the author guidelines state otherwise. Some journals ask that queries be sent to the Managing Editor. Write clearly and concisely. This is the editor's introduction to your writing. If your query is poorly written, the editor will assume that your manuscript will be the same quality. Include an abstract and, if asked for in the guidelines, an outline.

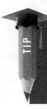

TIP

Remember that you cannot submit your manuscript to more than one journal. But you can send queries to as many journals as you want. Editors usually respond quickly to a query, so start with two or three of your top journal choices.

What to Include in a Query

- Brief description of the manuscript

- Why your manuscript is important—what does it add to the literature?

- Why you're qualified to write it

- A statement that it has not been published elsewhere

- Date when it will be ready for submission

- Approximate word count

- Your contact information

ALERT!

Don't send your manuscript in a query. It's presumptuous. The editor won't read it, and you will just annoy them. And you really don't want to annoy the editor!

Sample Query

Dear (Editor's name),

I am writing to ask if you would be interested in a manuscript on a research study of the effect of online resiliency training on short-term mental health outcomes in women survivors of intimate partner violence (IPV). Women who experience IPV are at higher risk of mental illness, including anxiety, depression, and PTSD. This study found that women who participated in a 6-week online resiliency training program had decreased mood disorder symptoms over the subsequent 6 months compared to the control group.

I am currently an assistant professor of nursing. The manuscript is a report of my dissertation research, which is included on the ProQuest Dissertation/Theses database. It has not been published. The manuscript is completed and ready for submission. It is 3,700 words, not including the reference list or tables. An abstract is attached.

Thank you for consideration. I look forward to your response.

Regards,

(Name)

(Title)

(Affiliation)

Submitting Your Article

You've taken your dissertation or scholarly project and reworked it into a well-written manuscript, chosen a few appropriate journals, and sent out some queries...and one is interested! Now it's time to submit.

All journals use an electronic submission process. There are three processes involved: typing information, electronically signing forms, and uploading documents. As the corresponding author, you are responsible for completing the process and making sure all your coauthors complete and sign any necessary documents. Journals have different requirements when it comes to coauthors. Some require that each author individually attests to authorship and complete disclosure statements, whereas others have the corresponding author complete all the forms in the name of all authors. If your coauthors are expected to complete their own documents, send them an email before you submit to let them know to watch for the documents.

Before you proceed, read the author guidelines. Each journal has specific requirements for submission. Table 9.1 is a checklist based on the most common requirements for submission. Journals may have different requirements, so read and follow your selected journal's guidelines. Then use Table 9.1 to make sure your manuscript is ready for submission.

ALERT!

Follow author guidelines! Ask any Editor-in-Chief what their biggest frustrations are and authors not following the journal's guidelines will be at the top of the list. Don't be one of those authors.

TABLE 9.1   Author Guidelines Checklist

My manuscript:
• Does or does not contain my or my coauthors' names as required by the journal
• Uses the correct formatting style
• Has the correct abstract formatting and headings
• Has a short running head that doesn't include author names
• Is the correct page or word count with or without references and tables/figures as required by the journal
• Does not exceed a maximum reference count if applicable
• Has the correct headings and subheadings
• Meets the criteria for the appropriate publishing standards and guidelines (such as SQUIRE or TREND)
• Has page or line numbers as required by the journal
• Does or does not have illustrations or tables/figures within the text (versus as separate documents) as required by the journal

Gathering All Components

Once you know that your manuscript meets all the guideline requirements, you're ready to gather everything you need to start the electronic submission process.

There are a number of pieces to a submission. Many journals require that you upload each piece as a separate attachment. For example, tables are uploaded in their own document, not as part of the main text. The same applies for figures or other illustrations. Make a checklist of all the pieces required by your selected journal, and create a separate document for each of them.

List 9.1 shows all the different pieces you need to have ready.

LIST 9.1 PRESUBMISSION REQUIRED COMPONENTS

Coauthor Information

Make sure you have up-to-date contact information, titles, and credentials for all your coauthors. It's best to send an email and ask your coauthors to confirm their information and how they want their name and credentials listed.

Cover Letter

The cover letter introduces your manuscript to the editor. Address it to the editor or Editor-in-Chief by name. Provide a brief one- or two-sentence summary of the article. Then include the following:

- **Prior communication:** Note if you've had any communication with the editor about the manuscript, such as a conversation at a conference or a positive response to a query you sent.

- **Previous or redundant publication:** Include a statement that the manuscript has not been published elsewhere. If your dissertation or scholarly project is on the ProQuest Dissertation/Theses database or an online repository, let the editor know. Also let the editor know if you presented the work at a conference and the abstract is published in conference proceedings.

- **Conflict of interest:** Let the editor know upfront in the cover letter if there are any potential conflicts of interest. (For more information on conflicts of interest, see Chapter 7, "Authorship: Rules, Responsibilities, and Legalities.")

- **Permissions:** Note whether you have obtained or are in the process of obtaining any needed permissions for illustrations, photographs, or other previously published materials included in your manuscript.

- **Corresponding author:** Provide the name and contact information for the corresponding author. Because this is your dissertation or scholarly project, you are the corresponding author.

Sample Cover Letter

Dear [Editor-in-Chief],

I am submitting the manuscript [Manuscript title] for consideration for publication in [Journal]. We met at the ENRS conference in March, and you encouraged me to submit a manuscript on this topic after viewing my poster, [Poster title].

The manuscript has not been submitted elsewhere, and the material has not been published in any form previously. The material is part of a larger study, and there is one publication that reports on other findings of that study. That article will be attached to the submission.

I am the sole author. I have no conflicts of interest to report. I would like to acknowledge [name and title] for her guidance with statistical analysis of the data.

Thank you for the time and effort in reviewing the manuscript.

Title Page

This includes the title of the manuscript, the names and affiliations of all the authors, and the contact information for the corresponding author. The title page is often where acknowledgements are noted.

Abstract

A well-written abstract provides a succinct summary of your article. After your title gets readers' attention, they will decide whether to access and read the article based on the abstract. There are two types of abstracts: structured and unstructured. The author guidelines stipulate which one to use. Also, take a look at the abstracts of articles similar to yours in the journal. Abstracts are usually 250 to 300 words, although some may be as short as 100 words.

Abstracts for research studies, quality improvement or practice change projects, and systematic reviews are usually structured. Typically, a structured abstract includes some or all of the following, with some variation among journals:

- Purpose or Objective
- Background
- Design
- Setting
- Sample or Participants
- Methods
- Results or Findings
- Conclusion
- Implications for Practice

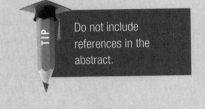

TIP

Do not include references in the abstract.

An unstructured abstract is most often used for clinical articles, concept analyses, or general review articles. It is usually one paragraph that provides a brief summary of the article, including the take-home message.

Sample Structured Abstract

Purpose: This study examined healthcare provider (HCP) perceptions of a rural community's IPV-related attitudes, beliefs, and barriers women face in getting help and compared their perceptions to the lived experience of women in the area they serve.

Methods: This was part of a mixed methods study that included a survey of rural HCPs' IPV-related knowledge, attitudes, beliefs, and behaviors and interviews with women who experienced IPV in the same region. This paper reports on open-ended questions about community factors at the end of the survey and compares the results to the lived experience of the women.

Conclusions: Overall, HCP perceptions were aligned with the experiences of the women. Blaming the victim was a strong theme in both providers' and women's perception of community attitudes, and both groups noted fear, shame, financial constraints, and lack of resources as primary barriers. HCPs also identified their own lack of knowledge and screening as primary barriers.

Implications for Practice: Along with better preparing healthcare providers to provide effective IPV-related care, we must address sociocultural factors that underlie the barriers women face.

Sample Unstructured Abstract

Obstetric fistula is a devastating complication of obstructed labor that affects at least two million women in the developing world, with an estimated 50,000 to 100,000 new cases annually. Research and safe motherhood interventions have focused on health education, training of skilled birth attendants, and alleviating poverty and barriers to access to skilled care. These are crucial components of safe motherhood; however, sociocultural factors beyond economics and availability of services may determine when and how women access services. Chief among these is gender power norms. Studies of other health problems have consistently shown that gender power imbalance has serious health consequences for women. Gender inequality and oppression of women are known to persist in regions where obstetric fistula occurs, yet little is known about the role of gender power imbalance related to obstetric fistula. This paper reports on a literature review of gender power imbalance in women in sub-Saharan Africa and Southeast Asia and its role in birth practices.

Keywords

Keywords are how readers find your article. They may be included with the abstract, or you may be asked to list them in a separate section of the submission. Choose these words carefully because they really are "key" to your article reaching readers who need the information.

Most journals ask you to list at least five keywords. Think about the words you would use to do a literature search for the information in your article. Make sure you list all the ways that people refer to the phenomenon or concept you're writing about. For example, in my articles on intimate partner violence, I include domestic violence, gender-based violence, and domestic abuse.

Nursing journals publish the keywords at the bottom of the abstract. Go through abstracts of some articles on your topic to get an idea of what keywords are used.

Manuscript Body

The author guidelines provide specific instructions on how to prepare your manuscript body. Journals vary in what they consider the manuscript body; for some it's just the main text and references, whereas others include the abstract, tables and figures, and other illustrations with the main text.

- **Author names:** In most cases, no author names should appear anywhere on the manuscript. This is to ensure blinded peer review.

- **Formatting:** Make sure you use the correct formatting style. Most nursing journals use APA. Do not go by what you see in their published articles; follow the author guidelines. Sometimes journals use APA for review and editing purposes and then reformat the manuscript in Chicago or AMA style for ease of reading and to save space.

- **Cover page:** Some journals ask for a cover page and have specific instructions for what to include on it.

- **Numbering:** Follow instructions about page and line numbering. Not all journals require line numbering, and those that do may specify that they start at 1 on each page or are continuous through the manuscript.

- **Reference formatting software:** Many journals insist that you *do not use* a formatting software program, such as RefWorks or EndNotes, for the references. It's difficult and messy for editors to work with during editing.

Artwork or Photographs

Photographs need to be a certain size and quality to maintain sharpness when they are reproduced. This is called resolution and is measured by dpi, or dots per inch. The standard dpi required for publication is 300 at the size at which the photo will be published. The smaller the photograph, the higher the required dpi so that the image doesn't lose sharpness with enlargement. Submit photographs in the correct format— usually as a TIFF, JPEG, GIF, or PNG. Do not submit a photograph as a PowerPoint slide or embedded in a Word document. Photos taken on a phone are not acceptable quality for publication. Include required permissions. (For information on what permissions are required for photographs, see Chapter 7.)

ALERT!

Do not repeatedly edit and save JPEG images that you plan to include with your manuscript. Every time you open, edit, and then resave a JPEG image, it loses data. In digital photography, data = quality. Make duplicates of the original image before editing a JPEG image.

COMMONLY ACCEPTED PHOTOGRAPHIC FILE FORMATS

- TIFF = Tagged Image File Format
- JPEG = Joint Photographic Experts Group
- GIF = Graphic Interchange Format
- PNG = Portable Network Graphic

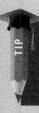

TIP

Some computer programs can add artificial resolution to a digital photo, but don't do it. It diminishes the quality of the photo instead of enhancing it. You lose detail and end up with an image that is muddy and pixelated. Once you artificially tinker with the resolution, the photo is unacceptable for publication.

Tables and Figures

Journals vary in how they want tables and figures submitted. Tables and figures may be submitted with the manuscript body or as separate attachments. When they are part of the manuscript body, they may be placed in the text where they would appear in the published article, or they may be included at the end of the manuscript on a separate page for each. If they are included at the end, you need to indicate in the text where they should be placed. All the information a reader needs to understand the table and figure must be included with the table or figure. Also, include a credit line if a table or figure is being reprinted or adapted from a previously published paper (see Chapter 7).

If you have additional tables or figures that are not part of the manuscript but could be published online as supplemental information, include them as attachments. Clearly mark them as supplemental materials, and make a note of that in the cover letter.

Permissions

It is your responsibility to obtain permission for the use of copyrighted materials, such as previously published tables or figures. In addition, make sure that you have permission for publication from anyone who is identifiable in photos. There may be specific forms for you to fill out, or you may be asked to provide a written statement that you have obtained permissions.

Forms

Authorship: You must complete authorship forms certifying that you and any coauthors meet authorship criteria. You may have to describe each author's specific contribution to the manuscript. As corresponding author, you may complete these and other forms for all the authors, or each author may have to complete her own.

Disclosure: You must complete disclosure forms related to any conflicts of interest for yourself or coauthors. A conflict of interest is any potential for personal gain that could bias the writing of the manuscript or the conduct of your research or project. This can be financial, such as earning fees to speak for a pharmaceutical company, but it can also be institutional, academic, or personal.

For more on permissions, authorship, and disclosure, see Chapter 7.

Additional Requirements

Institutional Review Board (IRB) Approval: Some journals require a copy of the IRB approval letter or, in the case of quality improvement projects, a letter from the appropriate IRB stating that IRB approval was not needed.

Clinical Trial Registry: If you've conducted a clinical trial, the clinical trial's registration information has to be included, usually in the cover letter.

Callouts: Some journals have you come up with your own callouts. Callouts are short sentences excerpted from the text of the article that are featured in large print in the article. Choose sentences that highlight key points. You don't have to repeat it exactly from the text; you can shorten it if needed.

EXAMPLE OF CALLOUT

Sentence in text.

> The belief that women can't make appropriate choices is not merely inaccurate; it also disempowers women and replicates the patriarchal attitudes that abused women are trying to escape.

Callout

> The belief that women can't make appropriate choices disempowers women.
> (Roush & Kurth, 2016)

Submit!

Go through the Submission Checklist at the end of this chapter to make sure you have everything ready. Getting through the electronic submission process can be time consuming, but having everything at your fingertips in the correct form will speed it up and save frustration.

The electronic submission system takes you step by step through the process. After you've uploaded your files, the system converts your submission to a PDF. You will be asked to review the submission; don't skip this step! I have caught errors in my manuscript at this step many times. If you see something you want to change, you can delete that version of your submission and upload a new one.

Now the waiting begins…. Be prepared, for it can take a long time to hear back. Some of this is due to the editor's reliance on volunteer reviewers who are busy with other obligations and often late completing reviews. If you don't hear anything after 3 or 4 months, send a polite email to the Managing Editor. If no Managing Editor is listed, send an email to the Editor-in-Chief asking for a status update. You can usually find the contact information for the Managing Editor on the website under the Journal Information tab or in the author's instructions.

In the next chapter, you learn what comes next when that decision finally arrives.

Step-By-Step

Submission Checklist

Cover Letter

- Have I addressed it to the Editor-in-Chief of the journal?
- Have I included a statement that the manuscript has not been published before?
- Have I included a statement that the manuscript has not been submitted elsewhere?
- Have I noted if the manuscript is from a dissertation or scholarly project that is on a repository, such as ProQuest or a program's website?
- Have I included any potential conflicts of interest or stated that none exist?
- Have I noted whether any needed permissions have been obtained?

Abstract

- Is the abstract the correct word count for the journal?
- Is it in the correct format—structured or unstructured?
- Have I removed citations from the abstract?

Keywords

- Have I included the required number of keywords (usually five)?

- Are the keywords the most likely search terms readers would use to find my article?

Manuscript

- Have I removed authors' names from the manuscript?

- Is the formatting in the correct style?

- Have I included page numbers and line numbers if required?

- Is the manuscript body the correct page or word count?

Tables and Figures

- Have I created separate documents for tables and figures if required?

- Have I included a placeholder for tables and figures that are not included in the body of the manuscript?

- Have I included a credit line for tables or figures that I reprinted or adapted from elsewhere?

- Do the tables and figures contain all the information the reader needs to understand their content (such as legends or keys)?

Permissions

- Have I addressed any permissions needed for figures, photos, or illustrations?

- Have I included any needed permissions from people who are identifiable or who appear in photographs?

Authorship and Disclosure Forms

- Do I have all the information I need from coauthors to complete authorship and disclosure forms?

- If individual forms are needed from each author, have they been completed?

- Am I being completely transparent in reporting any potential conflicts of interest?

- Have I disclosed all funding sources?

Reference

Roush, K., & Kurth, A. (2016). Intimate partner violence: The knowledge, attitudes, beliefs, and behaviors of rural health care providers. *American Journal of Nursing, 116*(6), 24–34.

10

GETTING A DECISION

This chapter addresses what happens when you get a decision back from the editor. It describes the different types of decisions and how to respond to each. Whether or not your manuscript is accepted, there is still work ahead—either getting ready for publication or using feedback from peer reviewers to revise and resubmit. Either way, persevere— you're almost there!

Finally, months later, just when you're about to give up hope of ever hearing word about your manuscript, you get a decision. There are three possibilities: accept, accept with revision, or reject.

If you have any concerns or questions related to the peer review or decision on your manuscript, contact the Editor-in-Chief of the journal. Most are open to a reasonable and respectful discussion on a decision. The Editor-in-Chief's goal is to have quality content for the journal. Starting a discussion about how you can revise your manuscript to meet that goal sometimes opens the door for resubmission, or it can give you new ideas for a different type of article related to your topic. Editors-in-Chief sometimes recommend alternative journals to submit to if your manuscript is just not a good fit for theirs.

Decisions

Accept: Congratulations! Celebrate, email your friends and family, and share the news with your colleagues. Then get ready for the next step in the publication process: working with the editorial staff to turn your manuscript into an article. (See page 174 later in this chapter, "Working with Editors.")

Accept with Revision: This is good news! It means the journal wants to publish your manuscript. Manuscripts are rarely accepted without revisions being needed. That is how a peer-review system functions to improve the quality of scholarly publication.

Reject: There is no getting around it; this outcome hurts. But do not despair. There are many reasons a manuscript may be rejected, including some that have nothing to do with the quality or importance of the manuscript. Just because this particular journal didn't want your manuscript doesn't mean that others will reject it. Most published authors, including me, have had a manuscript rejected on the first submission and then had it accepted elsewhere. Most journals offer you the reviewers' comments when they send you a rejection decision. Use those comments to strengthen the manuscript, and then send it out again. Do *not* let your manuscript disappear into a file on your computer, never to be seen again. Remember you believed in the importance of this work, and that hasn't changed just because your manuscript didn't fit the needs of one journal.

Common Reasons for Manuscript Rejection

The following list includes common reasons for a manuscript to be rejected:

- Not a good fit for the journal.

- Information is not new or timely or a similar article has been published recently by the journal.

- Lack of rigor in conduct of research or quality improvement initiative.

- Evidence of bias.

- No baseline data in a quality improvement initiative.

- Not adequately supported by evidence, or inappropriate sourcing.

- Information is superficial or too basic.

- Gaps in content.

- Ethical problems.

- Plagiarism.

- Poorly reported or flawed literature search strategy in systematic or integrative reviews.

- Poor writing.

- Does not follow author guidelines.

If you strongly disagree with the reviewers' rationale for rejecting the manuscript or believe there was bias in the reviews, contact the editor. Politely present your argument and ask that the manuscript be reconsidered. You must have specific details about why the editor should invest more time in the manuscript. For example, an author I worked with had a manuscript related to burns rejected because she included people who had Stevens-Johnson syndrome as burn survivors. Two reviewers thought this was an error that indicated that she was not well versed in the field of burn nursing. They were mistaken. These patients are treated in a burn unit and suffer similar sequelae. The author was allowed to revise and resubmit, and the manuscript was eventually accepted. (This is also a good example of the author having information she takes for granted that readers may need to understand the topic. It is also why getting feedback is so important. See Chapter 2, "Writing Well," for more on these types of details.)

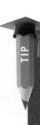

TIP

If the reviewers' comments and questions seem to indicate that there is a serious problem with the overall quality of the manuscript, consider hiring a Developmental Editor to work with you on revising. Editors can help with clarity, organization, and language, bringing out the importance of the work that poor writing may obscure.

FINDING A QUALIFIED FREELANCE EDITOR

- Ask your committee members for recommendations.

- Talk to senior faculty if you are in an academic position.

- Ask the editor of the journal if they can recommend editors they work with.

- Check the directory of freelance editors on the website of the Editorial Freelancers Association (https://www.the-efa.org).

Responding to Reviewers' Recommendations

The first time you read the peer reviewers' comments can be unsettling. First, do not take them personally. Second, sit on it. Do not make any changes until after you've let the recommendations sit with you a while—a few days at least and longer with a couple of rereads thrown in if you have the time. You will find that some of the comments you reacted against on first read now seem valid or even a valuable improvement to the manuscript. However, there may be some you won't agree with at any point, and that's okay. You don't have to make every recommended change, but you do need to provide a good explanation of why you are not.

ALERT!

Only make the recommended changes. Accept with revision is not an opportunity to make changes you thought of after you originally submitted the manuscript. Do not add information or rewrite passages unless you're asked to do so. And remember, you still have a page limit to contend with.

Follow the editor's instructions on how to make changes in the manuscript. You may be required to make the revisions in a different color so that reviewers can easily and quickly see the changes. You will also likely have to create a table that shows how you addressed each recommendation. This is where you should provide explanations for any recommendations you chose not to follow. Table 10.1 is an example of a table completed for an actual submission.

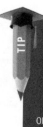

TIP

To make sure you address everything, print the reviewers' recommendations and cross out or highlight each one as you address it.

TABLE 10.1   Response to Reviewer Recommendations Table

Recommendation	Revision
Purpose of study is not clearly stated early on but is in the middle of the Background section.	The purpose is stated at the end of the Introduction—the last sentence of the third paragraph: Therefore, we conducted a study to determine the current IPV-related knowledge, attitudes, beliefs, and behaviors (KABB) of healthcare providers in the rural setting.
Sample 1. Need to define "providers and nursing staff"—do you mean physicians, NPs, PAs, and staff nurses? 2. What were the inclusion/ exclusion criteria?	1. Clarified on lines 91 to 93. 2. The inclusion criteria are stated on lines 91–94. There were no exclusion criteria. Everyone who met the inclusion criteria could participate.
Instruments 1. Describe each of the instruments used. Number of questions, psychometrics.	1. The description of the instrument is in lines 113 to 149. I added more information about the survey instruments. I moved information about the survey questions from the "Data Analysis" section to the "Instrument" section. I added information about psychometrics. See lines 125–133.
Data 1. Any differences in responses between various groups—frontline nurses, NPs/PAs, physicians? If not need to state that and explain data were collapsed. 2. 108 responded to the survey. Sample size varies across analyses—need explanation of why this is so.	1. The sample size was not large enough to look at differences between the groups. This is noted in lines 164–167. I don't think stating that data was collapsed is an accurate depiction of the analysis because it was never looked at separately to begin with. 2. This was an error. Thank you for picking it up. 108 responded and opened the survey, but only 93 completed it. The 15 who didn't complete it only answered the first few questions or did not answer any questions, so they were removed from the analysis. Other numbers vary because the questions did not apply to everyone (i.e., LPN or RN wouldn't answer questions about diagnosis). Changes were made on lines 170–172 to reflect this.
Limitations—sample size	I added "small" to line 360 and "other populations" to line 361.

Implications for practice need expansion—specifics for frontline nurses vs. NPs, MDs, classes in how to do assessment for IPV, how to know resources in community, etc.	Expanded. I reorganized so that implications are pulled out into one section as recommended by one of the reviewers. I respectfully disagree that implications need to be specific to frontline nurses vs. NPs, MDs, etc. The implications are applicable across roles. Also, the data was not analyzed by role, so it's not possible to say that one finding, and thus its implications, are applicable to one group.

Reviewer comments for:

Roush, K., & Kurth, A. (2016). Intimate partner violence: The knowledge, attitudes, beliefs, and behaviors of rural health care providers. American Journal of Nursing, 116*(6), 24–34.*

Peer reviewer comments should always be focused on the manuscript and not the author. Unfortunately, some reviews can come across as harsh or judgmental. Thankfully, these are the exception. If you do receive such a review, do not take it to heart. Try to just pull out the helpful feedback and let the rest go.

IMPORTANT

It is your responsibility as a writer to make sure that everything you write is understood *exactly* as you intended it to be understood. If reviewers misunderstand something, that is not their fault. It's a sign you need to revise for clarity. Remember, you have a lot of background information in your head, so you may be making connections that the readers aren't able to make based on what is written and what is missing. See Chapter 2 for more information on completeness of content.

Make sure you get the revised manuscript back to the journal on time. Remember to factor in time for each of the coauthors to review and agree to the changes. If you cannot meet the deadline, email the editor well ahead of time and request an extension. This is usually not a problem unless the manuscript is intended for a particular issue.

Finally, when you send the revision back, thank the reviewers for their time and expertise. Let them know you appreciate the improvements their recommendations have made to the manuscript.

Working With Editors

When your manuscript enters the editing phase, keep one thought uppermost—it's all about ending up with the best possible article. Remove your ego from the process. Even a well-written manuscript benefits significantly from a good editor. A good editor will make sure your manuscript says exactly what you meant it to say as clearly as possible.

Many nursing journals do not have an editorial staff but instead send accepted manuscripts to freelance editors. They may communicate directly with you or send the edited versions back to the Managing Editor who then communicates with you. Some editors set up an editing schedule with you so you know when you need to be available to respond to queries and check page proofs (these steps are explained further in this chapter), particularly if they are doing a substantive edit. In other cases, you may just receive an email with the completed edit with queries for your review and response.

IMPORTANT

There is a strict schedule for getting a journal issue ready for publication on time. It depends on everyone meeting deadlines. Once your manuscript enters production—which begins with the editing process—you need to meet the deadlines for each step of the process. Let the editor know if you are not going to be available to respond to queries or review pages at any time during the production process.

Types of Editing

There are different types of editing that your manuscript may undergo: developmental or substantive editing, copy editing, and proofreading. Most nursing journals do only copy editing and proofreading.

Developmental or Substantive Editing

This is the most extensive type of editing. The editor looks at the substance of the manuscript as well as the language and style, identifying gaps in content, eliminating redundancy, reorganizing for better flow, ensuring logical consistency throughout, and rewriting sentences for clarity and conciseness. If your journal does a substantive edit, don't be surprised if there are a lot of changes. However, a good editor retains the author's voice—but just makes it sound a whole lot better!

Some authors have difficulty with substantive edits, especially if they're used to having their work just copy edited. You may find yourself feeling defensive about changes to your work—after all, this is your baby you've sweated over and finally sent into the world thinking it was the best it could be. Remember: you are the content expert and the editor is the writing expert. Trust the editor's expertise. If there is anything that doesn't sit right with you, talk it over with the editor. Some changes are a matter of personal judgment about what works better.

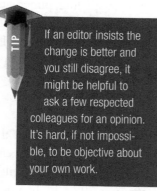

TIP

If an editor insists the change is better and you still disagree, it might be helpful to ask a few respected colleagues for an opinion. It's hard, if not impossible, to be objective about your own work.

Copy Editing

Copy Editors ensure a manuscript meets all accepted rules of grammar and style, including punctuation, spelling, capitalization, grammar, and sentence structure. They look at the language, including checking for jargon and redundancy. They cross-reference tables and figures for accuracy and consistency. They also fact-check and may check the accuracy of any math, such as calculating that percentages and numbers match up. (They don't do statistical tests.)

There is some overlap between a substantive edit and a copy edit. If the journal you're publishing with doesn't have a Developmental Editor work on your manuscript, the Copy Editor may make some content edits, reorganize for clarity or consistency, or note where there are gaps or problems with logic.

Proofreading

Proofreading happens after the manuscript has been laid out in its final form as an article. The Proofreader checks for any errors in grammar, spelling, punctuation, graphics, or formatting that were missed by the Copy Editor or introduced when the manuscript was converted into the article. The Proofreader checks page numbers, headings, and captions for photos and illustrations.

Queries

Queries are the questions that the editor asks you to clarify in the manuscript or simply to verify that a change they made is okay. The number of queries will vary—there may be as few as 3 or 4 or as many as 30 or 40. In a developmental or substantive edit, there will likely be a lot of queries. With a copy edit, the number will depend on how well written the manuscript is, particularly when it comes to clarity.

Don't panic if you open your edited manuscript and see a lot of queries. As you go through it, you will see that many queries are simply asking you to okay changes. Others may require more time, perhaps asking you to add information, recheck statistical results, or go back to your references to confirm sources. Tackle the queries one by one, and the process will quickly feel more manageable. Be thorough and clear in your responses, and stay on schedule so that the editing process isn't delayed. You will usually have one to two weeks to get your responses back to the editor.

List 10.1 gives you an idea of the variety of queries that you may encounter. They are actual queries taken from different manuscripts.

LIST 10.1   EXAMPLES OF QUERIES

1. Please provide version number for SPSS software.

2. Please check and confirm that changes to Table 1 are correct.

3. In Table 2, sentence ("The Web site …") correct as edited?

4. Underlined sentence added for clarity, OK?

5. Under Practice Implications you mention educational campaigns—such as?

6. On the survey, there's the acronym HHHN. What does that stand for?

7. These scores aren't reported in the tables, so please double-check and confirm.

8. I can't confirm 3-to-5 times greater in this ref; please confirm or provide alternate source.

9. Please cite refs to support this; or you can say "in our experience."

10. Please check all website addresses and confirm that they are correct.

11. Boyle & Jones 2006 is not in the Reference List. Please supply full publication details.

12. I think "viable" might be a better word choice than "relevant." OK?

13. Could you add a few words here about why this was done?

14. Can you perhaps provide a bit more context here? For example: What percentage of pts seen by nurses are victims of abuse, sicker because of disparities, etc.?

15. This section seemed long; I condensed it where it seemed possible without losing info. Please let me know if you disagree with any deletions.

Page Proofs

When the article is laid out and ready for publication, you'll get the "pages"—a PDF of the final version just as it will look in the journal. It's exciting to get pages and see the final transformation of your manuscript into an article. You'll be asked to carefully review them. You cannot make any major changes at this point; your task is to just check to make sure there are no errors. Usually there is a very short turnaround time for this—as short as a few days.

TIP

You may be tempted to just skim through the manuscript at this step. Don't do that. Read it carefully. Because editors aren't content experts, they can sometimes introduce an error when they make changes. This is your last chance to make sure the article reads exactly as it should.

The final step is author approval. You state in an email that you approve of the final version. The next time you see it will be in the pages of the journal. The wait isn't quite over yet, though. The production cycle for a monthly journal is about two months after editing is completed. Once you approve pages, it will be at least another month before it shows up in the print journal or online volume

Publication Ahead of Print

Some journals make a version of a manuscript available online prior to its publication date. Others publish an article online ahead of the print edition. They do this to facilitate more timely access to information because the length of time from submission to final publication can be so long. There are three versions of the article that may be available in press before the official publication date:

- Accepted manuscript that has not been edited

- Uncorrected page proofs that have not been reviewed or corrected by the author

- Corrected page proofs that have been reviewed and corrected by the author

In each of these versions, there may be some minor changes in the final published article, particularly with the unedited version. Once the article is published in a volume, the in-press version is removed.

For information about your rights to reproduce and distribute the published article, see Chapter 7, "Authorship: Rules, Responsibilities, and Legalities."

Step-By-Step

Key Points

- Patience. Peer review takes months.

- Do not let a rejection be the end of your manuscript. Revise and send it again.

- It's all about the manuscript—do not take reviewer comments personally.

- Address all reviewer recommendations.
- Meet all deadlines.
- Respect the editor's expertise.
- Answer queries clearly and thoroughly.
- Check page proofs carefully.

INDEX

Q

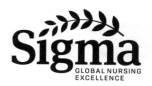

Sigma
GLOBAL NURSING EXCELLENCE

igma brings home more awards!

HECK OUT OUR 2018 *AMERICAN JOURNAL OF NURSING (AJN)* BOOK OF THE YEAR AWARDS

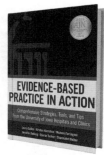

Evidence-Based Practice in Action
(9781940446936)

Second Place

Education/Continuing Education/ Professional Development category

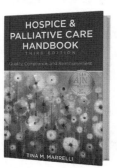

Hospice & Palliative Care Handbook, Third Edition
(9781945157455)

Second Place

Palliative Care and Hospice category

See Sigma's 2017 *AJN* Book of the Year Award recipients

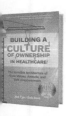

Iding a Culture Ownership in Healthcare

First Place

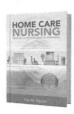

Home Care Nursing

Second Place

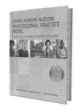

Johns Hopkins Nursing Professional Practice Model

Second Place

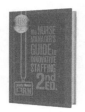

The Nurse Manager's Guide to Innovative Staffing, Second Edition

Third Place

Step-By-Step Guides for Nurses

A Nurse's Step-By-Step Guide to Writing a Dissertation or Scholarly Project, Second Edition

ISBN: 9781948057127

Karen Roush

A Nurse's Step-By-Step Guide to Academic Promotion & Tenure

ISBN: 9781940446882

Constance E. McIntosh, Cynthia M. Thomas, and David E. McIntosh

A Nurse's Step-By-Step Guide to Transitioning to the Professional Nurse Role

ISBN: 9781940446226

Cynthia M. Thomas, Constance E. McIntosh, and Jennifer S. Mensik

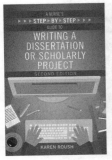
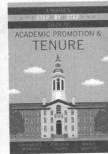
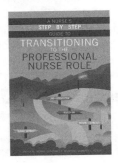

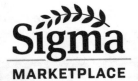